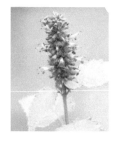
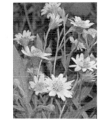
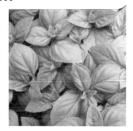

Adventures With Herbs
In Fairbanks, Alaska

By Virginia Damron and Marsha Munsell

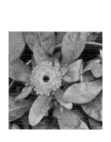
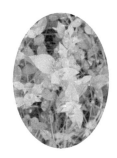
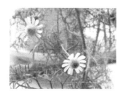

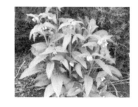
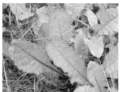
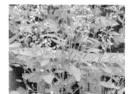

We are grateful for all the herbalists and users of herbs that have created the traditions and kept the knowledge that we can access today. We are especially grateful for the inspiration we received from Barbara Fay and all our friends in the Herb Bunch. Thank you,

Virginia and Marsha

Introduction

We can all connect to the past through the growing of herbs. Early evidence shows that ancient people grew many of the same herbs we do. There are 17th century records of arugula, basil, balms, chicory, cress, sages, hyssop, mint, and many others grown and used as salad herbs. Gardener's Dictionary written in 1731 by Phillip Miller instructed gentlemen in the art of herb cultivation. The early Greeks and Chinese also grew and used herbs for their healing constituents.

Can you imagine the smell of basil or rosemary just as our ancestors did, hundreds of years before us? Their problems were very like ours: soil, weeds, and many of the same tasks we have today. We love this continuity of planting and tending herb plants that have been around since any records have existed. We find comfort and joy in continuing a long tradition and hope you will too.

We began to learn about the use of herbs to enhance food from Barbara Fay, the Fairbanks herb master. She offered us opportunities to work and teach with her that fed our interest and led us further into this fascinating world. After Barbara moved, there was a void in the herb community and the group that had formed around Barbara's classes was struggling. We began to try to pull things back together to continue learning. We taught some classes here and there before we were asked to teach for a local greenhouse. We began teaching at Risse's Greenhouse on April 30, 2011. We have continued to teach three classes a year there and sometimes for other greenhouses and organizations. We have a great time and hope our participants do, as well as learn about herbs. Our repertoire has grown from culinary uses to include lotions, potions, and healing herbs. Marsha has had to drag me kicking and screaming into these new areas as I was only into culinary uses. Now, I find myself searching for current information about herbs for any and many uses.

Fairbanks Alaska can be a difficult environment in which to garden. We have bitter cold winters, hot summers, long dark spells, and long light spells. Rumor has it that herbs won't grow here, but as we move forward, you'll see that most herbs thrive here, and some are even perennial. Our hope for this book is that you will embrace herbs in their many uses, grow your knowledge of them and increase your interest in all things herbal in this northern climate. And that you can find as much passion as we have found. Now let's jump right into this journey. . .

All aboard!

Contents

Growing Herbs

Herb gardens can be as fancy as a maze or as simple as a square bed. They can be placed throughout your garden, as long as they are good companions to plants nearby. Herbs also grow really well in pots, placed in warm places.

Should you decide to plant a dedicated herb bed, you will need to do some preparation. First you will need to decide what you want to grow. Remember that a lot of the herbs we love are native to the Mediterranean areas of Greece and Italy and need a lot of sun. It is a good idea to draw a map of the bed as you want to plant it. Keep in mind the size of the adult plants and allow them room to grow. Try to keep the taller herbs from shading shorter herbs. Plant perennial herbs, such as tarragon and chives, where they won't be disturbed as you plant and harvest annual herbs.

Companion planting is a popular topic right now. However, it is at least as old as the three sisters planting of Native Americans. When the English arrived in America, the three sisters were corn, beans to climb on the corn and supply nitrogen to the roots of the corn, and squash to cover the soil, keeping it moist and to help prevent weeds. Now we have square foot gardening, which plants companions very close together and forest gardening, in which companion plants are intermingled to provide a mixed bed and create an ecosystem.

Organic gardeners use companion planting to avoid the use of chemical fertilizers, weed controls, and pest controls. In recent years, many certified organic garden products have appeared on nursery shelves, but it seems to us that it is better to use them judiciously and rely on natural methods for controlling bugs and disease.

Companion planting is like building a community. You get to design all the elements that make this community. The plants you choose and the amount of space available will determine the size of your community. We plant many of our herbs in the greenhouse with tomatoes and cucumbers. Basil, in its many varieties , is always there along with some flowers such as alyssum, gem marigolds or nasturtiums. Basil repels flies and mosquitos. Bee balm, chives, and int, reportedly, but untested, improve the flavor of tomatoes. Dill, on the other hand, stunts their growth, so should not be planted in our greenhouses but in the garden. Marigolds are great for preventing tomato horn worms and nematodes for tomatoes planted in the garden. We put Lemon Gem marigolds in the greenhouse as an added precaution with the hope to confuse the bugs and prevent damage to our other plants. Some other companion ideas are parsley with corn, and lettuce; sage with carrots, but not with eggplant; summer savory with both bush and pole beans, and thyme with onions and lettuce. There are multiple books and websites dedicated to companion planting. It is an interesting plan to follow.

Now back to building that herb garden. Find a warm spot that gets good light most of the day. Remove all the grass and weeds from the area and loosen the soil. Add organic matter, such as compost, until you have a quick draining soil mix. If you are doing a raised bed, you could also turn the sod over, cover it with weed block or ten layers of newspaper, and add soil and organic matter. Pile it high with organic matter and good topsoil. Then mix with a garden fork and level. Water thoroughly and wait for the weather to warm. Be sure to harden off your herbs before planting them outside.

Herbs can be planted in existing garden beds too. Add some compost, mix it in and again, when the soil is warm, plant your seeds or starts. Oregano, marjoram, thymes, shiso and sages will grow well outside in the sun. Basil can be a bit picky about where it wants to grow. Greenhouses and south facing spots seem to work best. In a rainy, cool year, many herbs will languish until a warm, sunny day comes and then they will take off. It is possible to have an instant herb garden, even in Fairbanks. The local nurseries carry a wide selection of herb plants, although you will need to nurture them inside until all danger of frost is past and some do even better if you wait until it is truly warm outside. The official first frost free day in Fairbanks is generally accepted to be

June 1. As our climate continues to change, this date may be somewhat fluid, but even that date is not always safe.

There is a lot of satisfaction in taking a tiny seed, planting it, tending it, and watching it grow until time to harvest. You can grow a much larger variety of herbs if you grow from seeds, however, some herbs must be bought as plants or rooted from another plant. Two such plants are French tarragon and lemon verbena. You can also buy one plant, get it growing then trim a healthy branch off, place it in water to root and pot a second plant up after the roots have established themselves. This can also be done with good success, using fresh herbs from the store. Snip off the hardened end remove a couple of the bottom leaves and place in water until they root. A pinch of rooting hormone will help this along.

Seed packets have a wealth of information on them, so be sure to read them. They will give you germination time so you can count back to a starting date, light requirements, and other information to help your seed get a good start. All 'you really need is seed starting mix, containers, water, seeds, good light, and time. If you are reusing containers, please douse them in a 10 parts water to 1 part Clorox or Lysol solution before using. We recommend a sterile starting mix unless you are very experienced in seed starting.

Containers can be anything big enough to hold the starter plant. Cottage cheese or yogurt containers, plastic pots, paper cups, 6 packs or flats – you get the picture. We have found that peat pots or the little mesh bags may not disintegrate in our cooler soils. You might consider removing them from around the root ball before planting. We have been told repeatedly by nurseries that the mesh bags do compost but have had plants languish, until dumped, only to find the roots bound by the bag. We now cut the bag or pull it off before planting. We suspect that in the greenhouses they do compost as the air, soil and water are warmer.

Years ago, a friend told me to put a layer of regular potting mix in the bottom 1/2- 2/3 of the container and then top with seed starting mix, so the roots have some nutrients to grab onto if I was slow to transplant. Dampen the soil and seed starting mixes until

3

a clump just holds together when you squeeze it. Fill your containers and place the seeds on top. Cover lightly with seed starting mix (unless seed requires light to germinate) and press lightly to insure good contact with the soil. Cover with plastic wrap, or for flats, the plastic dome covers that are available at nurseries. This will conserve moisture and help retain heat. Find a spot with good light. Place under a fluorescent or LED light fixture or near a bright window (not near the cold glass) until green shoots are showing. Water carefully. More plants die of over watering than under watering. Misting with a spray bottle works well. Plastic tops should be removed as soon as you see green. Herbs do best if they are about 2 inches below the light source as they grow. You must keep moving the light source up to keep from burning the young sprouts. Light fixtures hung on chains with S hooks make moving the light easier. 14-16 hours of light is fine, but they do need some down time too. When seedlings have two true leaves, they can be transplanted into a larger container until they are ready to face the big, bad world outside.

Plants may be fertilized with low nitrogen products such as fish or seaweed fertilizer when they have two true leaves. Damping off or seedling demise is a common problem, if you are not careful. It is usually caused by a pathogen called pythium, which is always present in all the sterile soil. Keeping all your materials as clean as possible is helpful. Stressed plants are far more susceptible to disease, so start with good seed from known sources and keep moist but not wet. Healthy plants can resist the pathogen.

While you wait for the weather to warm enough to transplant your herbs and if you haven't done so already, you can amend the planting area soils with compost or other organic matter. Herbs prefer a loose soil with a lot of organics to support their growth. If plants outgrow the starter pot and need to be transplanted before you get them into their summer spot, select a slightly larger pot (2 inches bigger) and fill with potting soil. Transplant the herb at the same depth as the original pot. Water well and keep in a protected spot for a couple of days before returning to full light.

Most herbs do well in pots if the roots have room to grow. Make sure the pot is sturdy and will not topple over from the weight of the plant. Felted bags are wonderful for herbs because they allow good drainage and air flow.

Now the fun begins! Your babied plant darlings will need to be hardened off gently to prepare them for the real world. Start by putting them outside in a sheltered area for one hour a day for a couple of days. Gradually move them into the sun and increase the time until they are in full sun for a full day. Now they are acclimated and ready to transplant into their permanent summer spot. Hopefully by this time the danger of frost is over, and the little darlings can flourish. Herbs, like most plants, require regular watering. Water deeply, don't just sprinkle. Let the plant's soil dry about an inch deep before watering. (That would be up to the first knuckle on your finger.)

A regular schedule of fertilization is a good idea. We suggest a fish or seaweed fertilizer at 50% strength about once a week.

You can begin to harvest as soon as the plant has a good root system and plant structure. Clip leaves or small sprig to use any time the plant can support further growth. Many herbs do much better when they are trimmed. You may start to trim plants as soon as they are 4-6 inches tall. This will encourage branching, thereby increasing your yield. Find a node above a leaf juncture and using clippers or scissors, cut the stem. Basil usually has two very small leaves at the juncture and greatly benefits from trimming. Do not use your fingers to pinch as this can crush the stem and do permanent damage.

The chart on the next pages will help you figure out what you want to grow and what to expect from it. We developed the chart from our years of experience in Fairbanks. Marsha lives in the hills where it is cooler in the summer and Virginia lives in town where it is warmer, so this represents our best guesses and our own experiences.

Culinary Herb Information
For
Fairbanks

Herb	Latin Name	Annual Biennial Perennial	Seed Start Date	Propagate By	Overwinter Indoors/Outdoors	Direct Seed	Reseeds	Degree of Difficulty
Anise Hyssop	Agastache foeniculum	P	Mid April	S	X		X	Easy
Basils	Ocimum basilicum	A	Mid April	S,C				Easy
Borage	Borago officinalis	A	Mid April	S			X	Easy
Calendula	Calendula officinalis	A	Mid April	S				Easy
Cilantro	Coriandrum sativum	A	Mid April	S		X		Moderate
Chervil	Anthriscus cerefolium	B	Mid April	S		X	X	Moderate
Chives	Allium schoenoprasum	P	Mid March	S, D	X		X	Easy
Dill	Anethum graveolens	A	Late April	S		X	X	Easy
Fennel	Foeniculum vulgare	A	Mid April	S, D		X		Easy

Herb	Latin Name	Annual Biennial Perennial	Seed Start Date	Propagate By	Overwinter Indoors/Outdoors		Direct Seed	Reseeds	Degree of Difficulty
French Tarragon	Artemisia dracunculus	P		C, D		X			Moderate
Lavender	Lavandula species	P/A		C, L					Moderate
Lemon Balm	Melissa officinalis	P	Mid April	S, C, D	X				Moderate
Lemongrass	Cymbopogon flexuosus	P	Mid April	S	X				Moderate
Lemon Thyme	Thymus species "Lemon Mist"	P		L, D	X	X			Moderate
Lemon Verbena	Aloysia triphylla	P		C, L	X	X			Difficult
Lovage	Levisticum officinale	P		S,D			X	X	Easy
Marjoram	Origanum majorana	P	Mid April	S, C					Easy
Mints	Mentha species	P	Mid April	C, D	X				Easy
Nasturtium	Nasturtium officinale	A	Late April	S			X		Easy
Nettles	Urtica dioica	P	Mid-April	S,D,C		X	X	X	Moderate
Oregano	Origanum species	P	Early April	C, L					Easy

Herb	Latin Name	Annual Biennial Perennial	Seed Start Date	Propagate By	Overwinter Indoors/Outdoors	Direct Seed	Reseeds	Degree of Difficulty
Parsley, Flat Leaf	Petroselinum var	B	Mid April	S				Easy
Rosemary	Rosmarinus officinalis	P	Late March	C, L	X			Moderate
Sage	Salvia officinalis	P	Mid April	S, C, L	X			Easy
Shiso	Perilla frutescens	A	Mid April	S		X	X	Moderate
Sorrel	Rumex acetosa	P	Mid April	S,D	X		X	Easy
Savory, Summer	Satureja hortensis	A	Mid April	S, C			X	Easy
Savory, Winter	Satureja montana	P	Early April	S, C, L				Easy
Sweet Cicely	Myrrhis odorata	P	Mid April	S, D	X	X	X	Difficult
Thyme	Thymus vulgaris	P	Mid April	S, C, D, L	X			Easy

Propagation Codes
S=Seed   C= Cutting
D=Division   L= Layering

Fairbanks Gardener's Winter Affliction

Catalog Fever is a locally occurring disease among gardeners. The disease is prevalent in January after the holiday rush when the garden catalogs arrive. Its symptoms are multiple order blanks from as many catalogs as possible and lengthy lists of catalog things we just must try this year. There is no known cure until the herbs come in! It does seem to mitigate the symptoms if you inventory stock on hand. It may also help to ask yourself the following questions and thus minimize the orders.

1. HOW MANY PLANTS DO I WANT? HOW MANY DO I HAVE ROOM FOR?

2. HOW MANY PLANTS CAN I TAKE CARE OF?

3. DO I KNOW ANYTHING ABOUT THIS HERB? OR DO I WANT TO LEARN ABOUT THIS HERB?

4. HOW MUCH OF THIS HERB WILL I REALLY USE?

USING HERBS

Herbs are used to add flavor and fragrance to food to enhance the taste, not dominate the dish. Some herbs impart a strong, very distinctive taste and some are mild and are used to finish and add color and flavor.

Herbs have an inordinate number of health benefits. They are a good source of micronutrients and flavonoids. Basil, for instance, has shown unique benefits in two areas of study, flavonoids, and volatile oils. It has anti-bacterial properties, anti-inflammatory effects and promotes cardio-vascular health. In addition to all that, it is an excellent source of vitamin A and manganese and a good source of copper, vitamin C, calcium, iron folate and omega 3s. If you want to explore the benefits of various herbs, we recommend whfoods.com for a start.

Strong flavored herbs can dominate a dish. Think about sage in turkey dressing. These herbs need careful consideration when

9

combining in a dish. Thyme with rosemary, sage, or marjoram will bring a nice note to your dish if used judiciously. French tarragon, with its strong licorice flavor blends well with basil but must be balanced. Savory is good with beans, but this is not one of my favorites, so I grow and use it sparingly. Marsha, on the other hand, loves it in soups and quiche. So she grows more. Oregano in Italian food and coriander (cilantro) in Mexican food are common flavors that dominate those ethnic dishes. Bay leaves mix with all the strong herbs and add a touch of floral taste to dishes with long cooking times. Another of the magical properties of herbs.

Accent herbs are exactly what that sounds like. They give a subtle background note. They combine well with any other herb and are usually a final addition to your dish. Parsley adds color and a nice fresh grassy hit to most any dish, but it is especially nice with chicken. Calendula will add a slightly bitter note and lots of color it added at the very last minute. Salad burnett with its cucumber flavor is nice with vegetable dishes or in salads.

We mentioned ethnic herbs above in the strong herb passage and there are a host of them out there. This is an area that is growing by leaps and bounds as we explore other cuisines. These herbs are specific to a dish and are hard to substitute. They are the foundation of the character of each dish. Some you may want to try are: Thai basil, Moroccan mint, Vietnamese balm, Epazote, Vietnamese coriander or red or green shiso (perilla). Most of these are becoming available either in seed or plants from local nurseries.

There are a myriad of herbs out there. Some you may not have tried but are interesting and mostly available. Borage with its sweet blue or white flowers, anise hyssop with its furry lavender spikes, lovage, sorrel, sweet cicely, sweet woodruff, mitsuma and nasturtium are some to try. We drink a bit of anise hyssop tea and eat borage flowers in salads for pure enjoyment.

The following will give you some hints for adding herbs to the foods you normally eat.

What Goes With What?

This is not a complete list but a starting place for trying different tastes to find what you like. Pick and choose. This list is suggestions, so don't pile everything on at once.

Vegetables

Asparagus: Lemon herbs, French tarragon

Beans: Marjoram, Savory, Basil, Bay Leaf, Epazote

Beets: Allspice, Bay Leaf, Cloves, Dill, Ginger

Broccoli: Dill, French Tarragon

Brussel Sprouts: Basil, Caraway Seeds, Nutmeg, Thyme, Marjoram

Cabbage: Dill, Caraway Seeds, Nutmeg, Chives, Thyme

Carrots: Allspice, Bay Leaf, Dill Ginger, Marjoram, Nutmeg, Thyme

Cucumbers: Basil, Shiso (Perilla), French Tarragon

Eggplant: Garlic, Marjoram, Oregano

Onions: Nutmeg, Oregano, Sage, Thyme

Peas: Basil, Dill, Oregano, Rosemary, Sage

Potatoes: Basil, Chives, Dill, Rosemary, Thyme

Green Leaf Veggies: Basil, Marjoram, Oregano, Nutmeg, Hot Peppers

Squash: Allspice, Basil, Ginger, Rosemary, Cinnamon, Nutmeg

Sweet Potatoes: Marjoram, Cinnamon, Nutmeg, Rosemary

Tomatoes: Basil, Bay Leaf, Oregano, Sage, Thyme

Salad Greens: Basil, Calendula, Chives, Cilantro, Dill, Marjoram, Oregano, Parsley, French Tarragon

Eggs: Basil, Dill, Garlic, Parsley

Fish: Basil, Bay Leaf, French Tarragon, Lemon Thyme, Coriander

Poultry: Basil, Cilantro/Coriander, Cumin, Marjoram, Sage, Thyme, Tarragon

Ground Meats: Oregano, Parsley, Sage, Savory, Thyme, Marjoram

Pork: Marjoram, Rosemary, Oregano, Sage, Thyme

Red Meats: Rosemary, Oregano, Tarragon, Thyme, Bay leaves, Coriander

Fruits (use herbs sparingly)

Apples: Thyme

Berries: Mint, Basil

Cantaloupe: Cilantro,

Cherries: Thyme, Basil

Citrus fruits: Mint, Thyme, Rosemary, Parsley, Tarragon

Cranberries: Rosemary

Fruit salad: Mint, Thai Basil, Sweet Basil, Tarragon

Honeydew: Mint, Tarragon, Thyme

Mango: Cilantro, Lemongrass, Mint

Pineapple: Lemongrass, Mint

Note: Some herbs in each category can be combined but combining all the suggestions for any one food at one time would overpower the essential flavor.

Dried or Fresh, How Much?

Which is best??

    A. What is available?

    B. Which has the most flavor?

    C. How much does it cost?

Herb flavor depends on:

    A. Fertilization while growing and growing conditions.

    B. Storage

    C. Age

    D. Preparation

Some herbs do dry well: Bay Leaf, Marjoram, Oregano, Rosemary, Thyme

Dried herbs should be stored in a cool, dark, dry place and used only if the fragrance and flavor are strong.

Fresh herbs can be loosely wrapped and stored in the produce bin of the refrigerator (except basil) or placed in a glass of water and placed in the refrigerator. Shelf life of fresh herbs is severely limited. Basil lasts longest in a glass of water, lightly covered with a loose bag, on the counter.

Another method of storing is freezing, and we will get into that later.

How much?

Use 2 to 3 times as much fresh herb to dried herb. (example: if the recipe calls for 1 teaspoon dried herb, use 1 tablespoon or 3 teaspoons fresh herb.)

My Herbs are Growing

Wow, we got through the hard part and now we have all this plush garden greenery, what are we going to do with it? This is where the fun begins. There are so many things to do that we get totally caught up in which to try.

A first step is always wandering out to the garden to select this and that for a salad. You can buy herb mixes at the store, but they've traveled a lot of miles and have lost a lot of their nutritional value before you get them. Pick as much of anything as you can use in one or two days.

Basil, Chervil, French Tarragon, Chives, Cilantro/Coriander, Parsley, and Lovage are always good choices for greenery. Add flower petals such as rose, nasturtium, begonia, marigold or

13

calendula for interest and color. This is only a small group of possibilities. Find your personal favorites and enjoy salad all summer.

You can really pick at any time, but for the most flavor, pick in the morning before the sun has had a chance to burn off some of the flavorful oils. This is also a good time to select herbs for your menu. We love to rub potatoes with olive oil, rosemary, thyme, salt, and pepper, then roast in a 425°F oven. Almost any herb will dress up carrots. Try melting a bit of butter and olive oil, add some dill and pour over cooked carrots. Yum! For a quickie pickle, try sliced cucumbers in a shiso vinegar for 30 minutes or more. This is a nice and unusual side for barbeque. The herbs provide endless solutions to providing tasty meals for friends and family.

Remember not to cut too much when you are gathering. Leave enough to support further growth and always snip at the leaf axil. This is the way to have fresh herbs all season. If growth gets ahead of you, harvest and preserve for later use.

Preserving is not rocket science with herbs. It is easy as can be. You can do slurries, pesto, butters, herb cheeses or just dry them for later. Stay with us and we'll show you how to do all of that later.

We plan our menus around what is fresh and available in the warm months. We both also have some dietary restrictions that play into what we put on our plates. Plan what works best for you. Look for the first asparagus in Spring. Brush it with olive oil, sprinkle it with lemon zest and French tarragon and roast in a 400°F oven until tender. What a treat after all the soups and stews of winter. Summer is the time for lots of salads. They may be grain-based or greens-based.

Grain bowls lend themselves to lots of herbs as they are pretty bland as a rule. Try a Tabbouleh with a big bunch of mint and parsley, then branch out and invent new family favorites. Green salads are always a hit. Pick colorful lettuces and add whatever you like. Any herbs that are growing, such as basil, mint, parsley, shiso, rose petals, nasturtium petals or leaves, or pansies will contribute bursts of flavor. Cucumbers, tomatoes, berries, nuts, celery, and carrots are all good possibilities to create a feast of flavors. Spring is also a good time to look for young or baby greens such as spinach or kale. These are great sauteed with a little garlic and the herb of your choice. Is there anything better that the taste of fresh spring peas?

As summer wears on, the repertoire of vegetables and herbs grow exponentially. Beans, carrots, cauliflower, beets, broccoli, and squash can all be changed from the mundane everyday food into something that excites your taste buds with a little pinch or two of compatible herbs. How easy is that?

SAVING HERBS

I've Got Too Much, Now What?

Preserving food has long been a means of storing food to ensure survival through the winter when nothing would grow. Modern times brought refrigeration, freezing and shipping improvements that relieved us of the need to preserve to survive. We now have food shipped to Alaska from all over the world.

Why, on earth would you spend the time and expend the energy to preserve your harvest? Well, we have several reasons for you to think about. You would always know where it came from. You would know if it is organic or grown with chemicals. You can get an early start by clipping, picking, thinning, or pruning. You can make teas and vinegars that you cannot buy or cannot afford. It is always fun to fill your pantry with your own homegrown food. AND maybe the biggest and best reason is that the closer to picking the greater the nutrients!

Compound butters are very expensive when you buy them at the grocery. One stick of butter, two or three tablespoons of herb and one teaspoon of lemon or lime juice is all it takes. You could add lemon, lime, or orange zest for extra flavor. Mix them all together and then shape or mold as you choose. Rolls are easy to manage and provide nice slices to top fish, meat, or veggies. Butter molded into shapes to match a holiday or simply as a decoration is a fun thing to do too. Butter will keep, in the freezer, up to a year.

We do what we call End-of Season Cheese, but you can do this any time you have bits of this and that to use up. Nothing ever comes out even in the garden, either too much or not enough, so this solves the herb problem. Measure your herbs (whatever combination you have) and add an equal amount of parsley. Chop them all together, then add an equal amount of Asiago, Kasseri, or a similar cheese. Put it all in the blender or food processor and pulse until well mixed. Put in containers and freeze for later use. You can also just eat it for your lunch! Use it on pasta, tomatoes, crackers, or sprinkle it on salads for a small protein hit and a huge flavor bomb.

Salts are an easy way to flavor food. It is also one of the oldest and surest methods to preserve fresh herbs. Dill, parsley, mint, rosemary, sage, thyme, cilantro, and basil are only a few that make wonderful salts. It is important to use good salt. Plain salt from the round blue box won't make the best salt, although it will work. However, if you are making the effort, then use coarse sea salt, Himalayan pink, fleur de sel, kosher or wood smoked. Wash 3 cups of loosely packed fresh herb and dry completely. You can let the herb air dry for a day or so to reduce the moisture. Remove stems from the herb and coarsely chop the leaves. Mix the herb and salt in a bowl. Mix until the mixture is uniform. You can use a blender or food processer by putting both herb and salt in the bowl and pulsing until you have a nice coarse salt, don't overmix or you will have salt paste. If the mixture is moist, spread it on a baking sheet and air dry. Stir once or twice to complete the drying process and to break up any chunks. You can also dry salt in a very slow (150/200°F) oven until it is dry. You can also make a quick herb salt by placing two tablespoons dried herb and four tablespoons salt in a blender. Pulse until combined and consistent in texture.

You can process more than one herb in a salt at a time. How about Herbes de Provence salt (rosemary, thyme, lavender and summer savory) or Italian salt (oregano, basil, rosemary, thyme, marjoram, sage, and savory) to speed up meal preparation? Salts can be used as rubs, sprinkles, or to finish a dish. Meats, potatoes, and popcorn are jazzed with a bit of herbal salt.

Sugars can be done much like salt, however the choice of herbs is usually a bit different, think mint, fennel, tarragon, basil, rosemary, lavender, anise hyssop or vanilla beans. You can also layer sugar and herb in a glass jar or closed container. Let sit for several weeks so flavor develops, or you can place in a food processor and mix until uniform. You can then store it in the freezer indefinitely. Use in teas, whipped cream, frosting, meringues or just sprinkle it on fruit. These suggestions are, to hopefully, get you on the road to experimenting to find what suits your palate.

It is possible to freeze fresh herbs. Leaves like basil or sage, lend themselves to cigar rolls. Lay out a piece of plastic wrap on a flat surface. Line up overlapping leaves across the width of the wrap. Fold over and start another row continuing until the herb is in a nice compact roll. Wrap the roll in foil, place the roll in a plastic bag and LABEL it. Be sure to label everything as they all look alike once they are frozen! To use, just open the roll and peel off the number of leaves you need and return the rest to the freezer. These are just like fresh herbs in cooking so add them at the end of the cooking time. They get very soggy when they thaw so use them quickly once they are out of the freezer.

One of our favorite ways to preserve fresh herbs is in a puree. We puree in olive oil, but any good oil will work. Oils preserve the aromatic oils in herbs that would dissipate in water. Use 1/2 cup good oil to 2 cups of fresh herb. Blend until mixture is a slurry. Pour into a plastic bag, flatten to remove air, and freeze, lying flat, on a cookie sheet. These will stand up nicely when solid, in a small basket in the freezer, making it easy to find the one you need. Break off the amount the recipe calls for and add at the appropriate time. Parsley puree is great for finishing a dish and adding that bright green splash. The little bit of oil will not affect the outcome or flavor of dishes.

Water purees or whole leaves in water are more for decorations than for flavor. Ice cubes with herbs look pretty in a punch bowl or drink but do little to enhance the flavor. You can infuse a liquid with an herb, make your drinks and then add your ice for a beautiful presentation.

Drying herbs is an age-old means of saving to use through the winter. There are dehydrators for sale everywhere or you can use a slow (150-170°F) oven until the herbs are brittle but not cooked. This will take up to 30 minutes or so. Don't raise the heat! You can also spread them on a sheet or drying rack until they are dry. Historical pictures show bunches of herbs strung across barns or still rooms to dry. Microwaving is fast but you must watch closely. Put small amounts of herbs on a paper towel, top with another paper towel and heat on high power in increments of 1 minute for 2 minutes then in 30 second increments. This can take up to 3 or 4 minutes. Leaves should remain green, so check often.

The easiest way to dry herbs is brown bagging. Water herbs the day before harvest, being careful not to splash the leaves with soil and allow the leaves to dry. Pick your herbs on large stems, if possible, throw them in a brown paper grocery sack, fold the top down twice and close the top with a clothes pin or staples and put in a cool dark place. Herbs will be ready to strip from stems in about a week. You can also spread herbs in a thin layer, in a cardboard flat to let passively dry. Always leave the herb leaves in as big a piece as possible before drying and when storing. Place herb in a container with a tight-fitting lid. Crumble just when using to preserve the aroma and flavor. Some herbs to try drying are marjoram, savory, chives, lavender, oregano, rosemary, mints, edible flowers, chamomile, and dill. Sweet Basil loses some of it flavor and aroma when dried. Thai Basil and the purple varieties dry pretty well.

Vinegars are an easy way to use excess herbs. Stuff a jar full of herb, pour over a good quality vinegar and let sit for a month. If the jar lid is metal, then cover the top of the jar with plastic wrap before putting the lid on. Strain and use in salad dressings, soups, and stews.

Nasturtium seed capers are handy to have in the refrigerator. Fill a pint jar with clean, dry nasturtium seeds, 6 peppercorns and about 2 cups of wine or rice vinegar. Seal and store for 3 or 4 weeks. Use as you would capers in any recipe. You can add a garlic clove, if desired.

Pesto can be made from many herbs. This is a mixture of herb, oil, garlic, cheese, and nuts that makes a paste used to enhance food. Cilantro, parsley, sage, and of course, basil are all good pesto herbs. Vary your oil, nuts, and herbs to find the combination that you like best. You can also make a vegan version with 2-3 tablespoons nutritional yeast rather than cheese.

Herbal mustard is having a moment right now. Make your own by mixing 1 1/2 cups mustard, 1/4 cup fresh finely chopped herb, and 1 1/2 tablespoons white wine vinegar. Cover tightly and refrigerate for up to three months. There are a multitude of mustards to try: stone-ground, Dijon, hot Chinese, or English. You can vary the vinegar or add a citrus zest, sweeten with brown sugar or honey, or flavor with garlic, chives, shallots, onions, horseradish and the chopped herbs to make it a signature of your culinary skill.

We do not recommend making herbal oils for consumption with fresh herbs, especially garlic oil. They are the perfect environment for botulism and other undesirable organisms to grow. Proper sterilization is just too difficult in the home kitchen. You can make an herbal oil for immediate use. Chop garlic and add it to oil, then brush bread with it and toast the bread for crostini or add herbs to a vinegar and oil dressing to be used within a few days.

Herb rubs seem to be a fad now as I type this. There are thousands of them online for you to try. Look for the ones that have ingredients you like or want to try. Make your own. Put some on your next piece of meat or sprinkle some on a bowl of vegetables. They add a spark of interesting flavor to your dish that will draw oohs and aahs.

Herb teas are great for relaxing and enjoying a respite from the whirl of daily activities. Anise hyssop, lemon balm, lavender, lemon thyme, lemon verbena, ginger, lemongrass, chamomile and all the mints and scented geraniums are good choices for tea. You can, of course, use any herb that you prefer or a combination of herbs that suit your palate. Use 1 teaspoon of crumbled dried herbs or 1 tablespoon of fresh herbs in a tea ball, bag, or sieve to start. Pour 1 cup boiling water over the herbs and let steep for 8 to 15 minutes. Herbs can become bitter if steeped too long. You may have to adjust the quantity of herb to make your tea stronger or weaker. Please experiment to find your personal preference.

Lemonade made with mints or lavender is extra special for guests. It is easy to make and is very refreshing. Steep 2 tablespoons of herb in 1 cup boiling water for 10 minutes, let cool and add to 1/2 gallon of lemonade. Try that at your next patio gathering.

You can dress up ciders with the addition of compatible herbs. Add a handful of lemon-flavored herbs to boiling apple juice or cider. Steep off heat for a few minutes, strain and enjoy.

You get lemon water in many high style restaurants today. You can add herbs like mints or lemon verbena to water and improve the taste and your enjoyment.

The next few pages will have some recipes for you to try. They are easy and use ingredients easily found in our grocery stores or farmer's markets. Get started on an herby life

RECIPES

Cream Cheese with Herbes de Provence

1-15 oz. pkg. cream cheese

1 ½ -3 Tbsp. cream or milk

1 garlic clove crushed and minced very fine

½ tsp. herb or white wine vinegar

1 tbsp. Herbes de Provence

¼ tsp. salt

Pinch of cayenne pepper

Cream the cheese with milk/cream until spreadable. Add Herbs de Provence, garlic, salt, cayenne, and vinegar. Blend well, cover tightly, and refrigerate for at least 2 hours. Taste and adjust seasoning. Flavor improves after a day and stores for 4 or 5 days refrigerated. Serve with crackers or as a spread for sandwiches.

Quinoa Salad

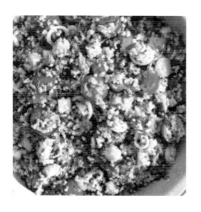

1 cup nuts, almonds, or pine nuts

3 Tbsp. fresh mint, chopped

1 or 2 tomatoes, chopped

2 Tbsp. lemon juice

1 cup fresh parsley, chopped

2 cups frozen petite peas

3 tbsp. olive oil

1 tsp. garlic salt

Salt and Pepper to taste

2 cups quinoa, cooked

Combine quinoa, nuts, mint, parsley, scallions, peas, and tomatoes in a large bowl. In a separate bowl, whisk together olive oil, lemon juice, and garlic salt. Pour over quinoa mixture. Gently toss dressing into quinoa mix. Season to taste with salt and pepper. Chill for at least 15 minutes. Toss gently before serving to recombine dressing with quinoa. Taste and adjust seasoning, if needed.

Hungarian Mushroom Soup

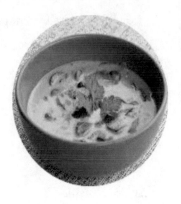

2 cups chopped onion

1- 1/2 to 2 lbs. mushrooms, sliced

1 tsp. salt

2-3 tsp. dried dill or 2-3 tbsp. of fresh

1 tbsp. mild paprika

2 tsp. lemon juice

3 tbsp. flour

2 cups vegetable broth or chicken broth

1 cup milk

Black pepper to taste

½ cup sour cream (can use low-fat)

2 tbsp. butter

Melt butter in kettle or Dutch oven. Add onions, and sauté over medium heat for about 5 minutes. Add mushrooms, salt, dill and paprika. stir well and cover. let cook for about 15 minutes, stirring occasionally. Stir in lemon juice. Gradually sprinkle in the flour, stirring constantly. Cook and stir another 5 minutes or so over medium heat. Add vegetable broth, cover, and cook about 10 minutes, stirring often. Stir in milk; add black pepper to taste. Check to see if it needs more salt. Whisk in the sour cream and heat very gently. Don't boil or cook it after this point. May be held on very low temperature (crockpot). Serve hot. May be garnished with fresh basil or parsley.

Serves 4 or 5.

Gremolata Rubbed Roast Beef

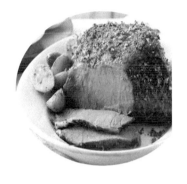

1/2 cup chopped fresh parsley

2 tbsp. fresh thyme leaves

1/2 head garlic

1 tbsp. olive oil

1 tbsp. salt

Zest of 1 lemon

For the Beef:

2 tbsp. olive oil

1 eye of round roast (4 lb.)

salt

For Gremolata:

Salt and sear roast in the olive oil. Combine all gremolata ingredients in a resealable bag.

Crush the garlic cloves with the herbs with flat side of knife or meat mallet. Mix. Season roast with salt and rub with gremolata.

Roast at 250 degrees for 2 1/2 hours or until roast reaches 130-135 degrees on meat thermometer. Allow roast to rest for 15 minutes before carving.

Prosciutto Wrapped Halibut With Sage

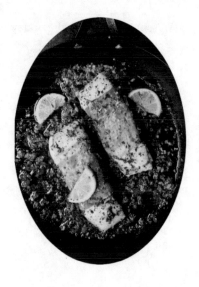

2 large lemons

6 1-inch thick skinless halibut filets

Kosher salt & fresh ground pepper

36 fresh sage leaves

6 thin slices Prosciutto

6 tbsp. unsalted butter

Position a rack in the center of the oven and heat the oven to 400°F.

Slicing crosswise, cut six 1/4-inch rounds from the center of one of the lemons. Repeat with the other lemon. Squeeze the juice from the ends of the lemons and set aside. Arrange the lemon slices (slightly overlapping) in pairs on a rimmed baking pan. Season fish with salt and pepper.

Place 2 sage leaves on each filet and then wrap in prosciutto (should form a belt covering sage but leaving ends of fish exposed.) Lay each filet on the lemon slices. Bake until the fish is cooked through and flakes easily (15 to 20 minutes).

While fish is cooking, melt the butter in a skillet over medium low heat. Add the rest of the sage leaves and cook turning until sage is crisp and the butter begins to brown (about 7 minutes). Add the lemon juice and season to taste.

Arrange filets on lemon slices on plates. Pour juice (if any) from fish into butter sauce. Reheat if necessary. Spoon sauce and sage leaves over filets and serve.

Asian Inspired Salmon in Foil

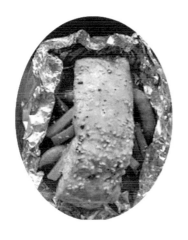

1/4 cup honey

3 cloves garlic, minced

2 tbsp. soy sauce

1 tbsp. rice vinegar

1 tbsp. sesame oil

1 tbsp. fresh grated ginger

1 tsp. sriracha (optional)

Dried, crumbled shiso (optional)

2 pounds Salmon

1 large carrot, julienned

8 oz. snow peas

8 oz. fresh mushrooms, sliced

Green onions, chopped

Sesame seeds

Salt and pepper

Mix honey, garlic, soy sauce, rice vinegar, sesame oil, ginger, sriracha, possibly shiso, and pepper to taste in a small bowl. Tear foil squares to fit salmon pieces. Place on a baking sheet. Put salmon on foil, top with mushrooms, carrots, and snow peas. Drizzle sauce mixture over packets. Fold up sides of foil and seal. Bake 15 to 25 minutes at 375 degrees. Depending on thickness of salmon. Open packets and garnish with green onions, and sesame seeds, if desired. Serve immediately.

Easy Chicken Piccata

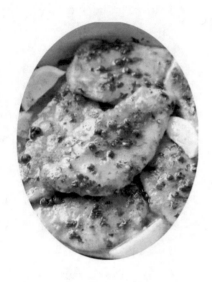

2 large lemons

1 bag chicken tenders

1/2 cup all-purpose flour (may be gluten free)

4 tbsp. olive oil

1 small shallot, minced or 1 small garlic clove, minced

1 cup chicken stock

1 tbsp. drained small capers**

1 tbsp. unsalted butter, softened

2 tbsp. fresh parsley, minced

2 tbsp tarragon, minced

Place oven rack in the middle, set large heatproof plate on rack and preheat to 200°F. Halve one lemon, pole to pole. Trim ends from 1/2 and cut crosswise into slices 1/8 to 1/4 inch thick; set aside. Juice remaining 1/2 and whole lemon to obtain 1/4 cup juice: reserve. Sprinkle both sides of chicken tenders with salt and pepper. Put flour in a shallow bowl and coat one tender at a time, shake to remove excess flour. Heat heavy bottomed skillet over medium high heat until hot, about 2 minutes; add 2 tbsp. olive oil and swirl to coat pan. Drop chicken tenders into pan and cook until browned on both sides, about 2 1/2 minutes per side. Transfer tenders to heated plate in oven. Add remaining oil and sauté remaining chicken tenders. Remove from heat to oven plate.

Add shallot or garlic to skillet and sauté over medium heat until fragrant. Add stock and lemon juice, increase heat to high and scrape skillet bottom with a wooden spoon to loosen browned bits. Simmer until reduced to about 1/3 cup (about 4 minutes), add lemon slices, capers and tarragon and reduce again to 1/3 cup. Remove pan from heat and swirl in butter until butter melts and thickens sauce, swirl in parsley. Spoon sauce over chicken and serve immediately. May be held at low temperature for 2 hours in oven or slow cooker.

Herb Substitution suggestion:

Replace tarragon with one of the following: 3 tbsp. coarsely chopped basil, 2 tbsp. finely snipped chives, 1 tbsp. coarsely chopped fresh marjoram or Italian oregano, 2 tbsp. coarsely chopped fresh spearmint or 2 tsp coarsely chopped fresh English or lemon thyme.

* *May use nasturtium capers

Greek Chicken Pizza

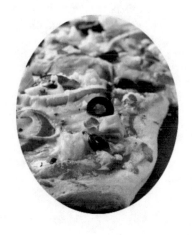

1 cup boneless, cooked chicken, shredded

5 oz. spinach

1/2 cup yogurt

1 1/2 tsp lemon Juice

4 1/2 tsp. chopped fresh dill or basil

1 chopped green onion

1 tsp. chopped garlic

¼ cup sliced red onion

½ cup sliced olives

1 cup shredded Mozzarella cheese

1/3 cup Feta cheese crumbles

1 thin crust pizza shell

Preheat oven to 425°F. Microwave spinach with 1/2 cup water for 1 1/2 minutes. Drain and (when cool) squeeze dry. Season with salt and pepper. Mix yogurt, lemon juice, dill, chopped green onions and garlic until combined. Spread yogurt mix on pizza crust, top with spinach and sliced red onion. Add chicken, feta cheese and mozzarella cheese. Bake on bottom rack of oven 10-15 minutes until golden and bubbly. Makes 8 slices.

Fresh Tomato Spaghetti

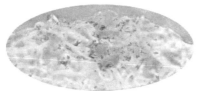

1/4 cup sliced almonds

3 tbsp. butter

1 cup whole wheat panko

1/3 cup flat leaf parsley, finely chopped

2 tbsp. fresh thyme, chopped

salt & pepper

3 pints cherry or 5-6 tomatoes

3 tbsp. olive oil

6 cloves garlic, chopped

1 lb. spaghetti

1 lemon zested (1 tsp.) and juiced (about 1/4 cup)

Extra Virgin olive oil for drizzling

1 cup grated Parmesan-Reggiano

Bring large pot of water to boil. Heat skillet and toast almonds. Finely chop cooled almonds.

Melt butter in skillet. and brown panko (about 2 minutes). Put panko, almonds & herbs in a bowl and mix thoroughly. Halve cherry tomatoes, if using. For larger tomatoes, cut x in bottom and plunge into boiling water (about 30 seconds) and then place in ice water to cool and stop cooking (about I minute). Dry, peel and chop tomatoes. Bring water back to boil. In a large skillet heat olive oil over medium heat. Add garlic (soften but don't brown). Add tomatoes and season to taste. Salt the water and cook pasta.

Remove 1/2 cup cooking water and then drain pasta. Add lemon zest & juice, basil, pasta and cooking water to tomato sauce.

Drizzle with Extra Virgin Olive Oil and toss to combine. Check and adjust seasoning. Serve in shallow bowls topped with panko/almond mix and shredded cheese.

*Works with any tomato. Yellow tomatoes are excellent.

Creamy Cauliflower Soup with Gemolata

Gremolata is a classic Italian garnish that will keep up to a week in the refrigerator. You can also use it to garnish pasta, stews and bean dishes (especially white beans).

Gremolata:

3 tablespoons chopped parsley

3 cloves garlic, chopped

1 tablespoon lemon zest

Creamy Cauliflower Soup:

2 tbsp. olive oil

1 medium-sized onion, sliced (about 1 cup)

1 large clove garlic, sliced

1 medium-sized apple, peeled, cored, and diced

1 head cauliflower, cut into florets (about 5 cups)

2 teaspoons lemon zest

½ teaspoon sugar

1/8 teaspoon nutmeg

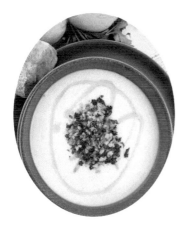

To make Gremolata: Combine parsley, garlic and lemon zest in small bowl and set aside.

For soup: Heat oil in large saucepan over medium heat. Add onion, garlic, and apple. Sauté about 7 minutes or until soft. Stir in remaining ingredients, cooking 2 more minutes. Add 4 cups water and bring to a boil. Reduce heat to medium-low and simmer 15 to 20 minutes or until cauliflower florets are very tender. Puree with immersion blender or in small batches in a blender or food processor. Return soup to saucepan and return to simmer. Season to taste with salt and pepper. Ladle into bowls, topping each serving with 1 tablespoon of gremolata.

Chimichurri for Meats or a Dip

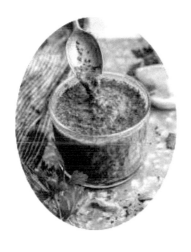

½ cup fresh parsley, stemmed

1 ½ cups cilantro

½ cup onion

3 tbsp. fresh oregano

3 cloves garlic

1 tbsp. lime juice

1 tbsp. red wine vinegar

½ tsp. ground cumin

¼ tsp. salt

¼ teaspoon pepper

¼ teaspoon ground ancho chili or to taste

½ cup olive oil

Place everything in a food processor and process to an almost smooth consistency. Leave some texture. Serve over meats or as a dip with crackers.

Salsa Verde for Steak

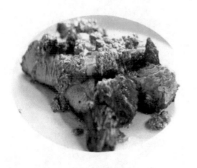

½ shallot, peeled

1 clove garlic, peeled

1 ½ tsp. capers, drained

1 anchovy fillet, rinsed and patted dry

2 tsp. fresh rosemary

2 tsp. fresh thyme

1 cup lightly packed parsley

1 tbsp. coarsely chopped walnuts

2-3 tbsp. red wine vinegar

½ tsp. black pepper

½ tsp. salt

½ cup olive oil

Place everything except olive oil in a food processor and process until finely chopped. Add oil and process until well blended. Serve at room temperature.

Lemongrass Chicken Soup

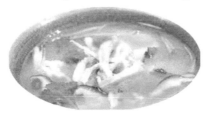

Simmer 2 quarts of homemade or store-bought chicken broth with 1/3 cup coarsely chopped lemongrass and 2-3 cloves garlic for 30 minutes. Strain lemongrass and garlic. Add whatever vegetables you desire and simmer until they are cooked. Add cooked chicken, cooked rice (if desired), salt and pepper to taste, and heat through. Serve warm with a sprinkle of fresh cilantro

Shiso Lemonade

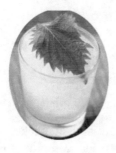

10 cups water

6 oz. red/purple shiso (perilla) leaves

1 cup lemon juice

1 to 2 cups sugar to taste

Bring 2 cups water to boil. Add shiso leaves and remove from heat. Steep 15 minutes. Strain and add sugar. Stir to dissolve sugar. Add lemon juice and 8 cups water. Store in the refrigerator. Serve over ice. Makes a lovely refreshing drink with added nutrients.

*Shiso, also called Perilla, may be red, purple, or green.

Shortbread with Lavender or Rosemary

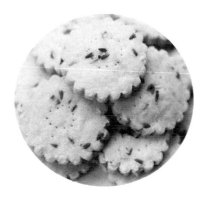

1 cup unsalted butter

½ cup sugar

1 ½-2 teaspoons finely chopped rosemary or lavender

2 ½ cups gluten free flour mix or regular flour

1 teaspoon vanilla

Cream butter, sugar, and herb. Add flour of choice and mix well. Roll out to about ½ inch thick. Cut into rounds or squares. Bake at 350°F until lightly browned, about 8-10 minutes.

Lemon-Ginger Shortbread

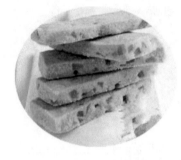

2 ½ cups gluten-free flour

1/2 cup almond meal

1/2 tsp. salt

1/2 lb. unsalted butter, softened

1/2 cup firmly packed brown sugar

1/3 cup finely chopped crystallized ginger

1/2 tsp. pure vanilla extract

1 tbsp. lemon zest

Sweet rice flour for dusting

Combine rice flour, sweet rice flour, almond meal, xanthan gum, and salt. Whisk together. Combine butter, and sugar and beat at low speed to combine. Increase mixer speed to high and beat 3-4 minutes or until light and fluffy. Add ginger, vanilla and zest and beat for 1 minute. Add flour mixture to butter mixture, slowly and beat until stiff dough forms. Wrap dough in plastic wrap and press into a pancake. Refrigerate 1 hour, until firm. May refrigerate up to 2 days. Preheat oven to 350°F. Line 2 baking sheets with parchment or baking mats. Dust sheet of waxed paper and rolling pin with sweet rice flour. Roll to ½-inch thickness and cut into rectangles about 4x1 inches. Transfer to baking sheets. Reroll to use excess dough (may need to be chilled for 15 minutes). Bake 12-15 minutes until edges are brown. Cool two minutes on sheet and then transfer to a rack until completely cool. Makes about 2 dozen.

Rosemary & Pine Nut Cookies

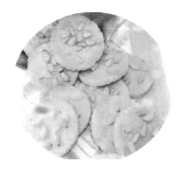

1 1/2 cups flour

1/2 tsp baking soda

1/4 tsp. salt

3/4 cup sugar

1 1/2 tsp. chopped fresh rosemary

1/2 cup pine nuts, toasted

3/4 cup unsalted butter

I large egg

½ tsp. pure vanilla extract

Combine flour, baking soda and salt until well mixed. Set aside. Pulse sugar and rosemary in a food processor until finely chopped. Transfer to mixer bowl. Put all but 2 tbsp. of pine nuts in food processor and process until finely chopped. Add the softened butter to the sugar mixture and beat on medium speed until light and fluffy (about 2 minutes). Reduce mixer speed to low and add egg and vanilla, beat until combined. Add chopped pine nuts and then the flour mixture. Mix until dough absorbs the flour and comes together. Turn the dough out onto a piece of plastic wrap and shape into a log. 2" x 11". Refrigerate for 2 hours. Preheat oven to 350°F and place rack in center of oven. Slice dough into rounds 1/4 to 1/2 inch thick. Sprinkle cookies with 2 tablespoons of whole pine nuts and gently press into dough.

Place on cookie sheets about 1 1/2 inches apart. Bake 1 sheet at a time until set and edges are lightly browned (10-12 minutes) Cool 10 minutes. Remove from cookie sheets and cool completely on racks. Serve or store in airtight container up to five days. Makes 30 cookies.

HEALING HERBS

We want to be sure that you understand that we have no special qualifications to practice any form of medicine. The information that we are providing came from several trusted herbalists' websites, books and from our own experience.

We believe that this is the latest and best data available to us right now. We cannot of course, cover every single healing herb, but we have chosen the ones with current studies and testing as well as some that will grow in Fairbanks.

Chinese Traditional Medicine, Ayurvedic, and Egyptian healers have depended on herbs for millennia. The German E Commission has studied and approved a large pharmacopeia of herbs that are useful for healing. Until recently, very little research was done in the USA. Now interest in the possibilities of healing herbs, has blossomed and studies and books have proliferated. We encourage you to thoroughly research any herb you plan to use for healing before jumping in. Herbs work differently for each of us. Nothing is ever a sure thing. I have a friend who swears by echinacea for colds. I am allergic to it and cannot use it or any product that contains it.

There are products and herbs you should avoid if you are pregnant. There are a multitude of herbs that can interfere with your prescription drugs. There are herbs that children should not have. There are herbs that are highly poisonous when ingested but that can be used topically. These cautions are to remind you that careful study and consideration needs to accompany any use of herbal medicines.

Herbs are not like pharmaceuticals. They have many actions on many parts of the body and affect different people in different ways. Herbalists don't think of what herb will cure a cold, they ask what kind of cold, what are the basic attributes of the person, is it wet or dry?

There are many things to consider when using herbs.

It is easy to get led down the garden path with all the hype for the wonderful cures available that the government won't let

41

you have etcetera... Please consider that, whether herbal or pharmaceutical, all medicines may have different effects on different people and some can be unexpected. Have we said investigate?

There are charlatans among us!

Teas & Infusions

Teas and infusions are quick and easy ways to prepare medicinal herbs. They are simply herbs and water. They can be used for poultices, drinking, or spraying on topically, or they can be concentrated into a syrup. Dry teas (combinations or single herbs) will keep 1 to 4 years in a cool dark place if sealed in an airtight container.

To make a tea or infusion, combine herb and boiling water according to your recipe amounts. Cover, steep for at least 10 minutes and strain to remove tea leaves. Cool as necessary before using.

For a syrup, make a strong herb tea. After steeping, strain and add up to 1 cup of honey and heat gently to 105-110 degrees. Pour syrup into sterilized bottle or jar.

To make a poultice, soak a hand towel in strong tea and place on the affected area.

Tinctures

Tinctures are simply infused extracts. The vanilla extract that you use in baking is similar to a tincture. Tinctures are usually made with an alcohol base, but they can also be made with apple cider vinegar or vegetable glycerin. Shelf life of an alcohol tincture is 7 to 10 years, with glycerin up to 3 years and with apple cider vinegar, 6 to 12 months. Both glycerin and apple cider vinegar tinctures should be refrigerated for storage and work with a limited number of herbs. The most commonly used alcohol is 80 proof vodka, but other high alcohol content liquors may be used. Generally, a tincture is 1 part herb to 2 parts liquid. If the herb swells above the liquid, top off with a little more. Always sterilize all utensils and equipment when making a tincture.

To make a tincture, put measured herbs in a sterile glass jar. Fill jar with appropriate amount of alcohol, glycerin, or apple cider vinegar. Generally the liquid should cover the herb. Put on a tight- fitting lid. You can place a layer of wax paper between the lid and jar to prevent oxidation of the lid. Place in a cool, dark area for 6 to 8 weeks, and shake weekly. If alcohol evaporates, top off the jar. To decant: put a piece of cheesecloth or muslin over a funnel in the mouth of a sterile jar, pour tincture through cheesecloth to remove herbs. Squeeze the fabric to extract as much as you can of the herb's properties. Your tincture is now ready to use.

Herbal Oils

Oils may be used alone but are most often the base for a salve or ointment. They are easy to make and handy to have available.

The usual oil ratio is 1 part herb to about 7-10 parts oil. We usually use 1-ounce dried herb to about 7 ounces of oil and go from there. Oils are a personal choice in that olive, almond, coconut, and Jojoba are all good choices.

Different oils are good for different skin types. If you have normal skin, go for oils like jojoba, extra virgin olive oil, and coconut which are not heavy on the skin. For dry skin oils like argan, grapeseed, apricot kernel, extra virgin, almond, and rosehip oils work best. Grapeseed oil also works good with oily skin.

Make sure that your herbs are thoroughly dry as any dampness will cause mold.

The warm quick method: Place the herb in the bottom of any device that will hold heat at 105 to 110 degrees. Heat at the lowest possible setting for 3-6 hours. Watch that the heat stays in that 105-to-110-degree range. Excess heat will compromise the herb constituents. Allow to cool completely. Strain through unbleached muslin into a clean sterile bottle. Squeeze as much out of the cloth as you can to extract all the good stuff.

43

Small dip slow cookers, yogurt makers, multi-cookers, or similar appliances have lower heat settings and may be easier to control.

The cold, long term method: place the herb and oil in a sterile jar and place it in a place where you will remember to shake it occasionally. Let it sit for 4-6 weeks before straining and decanting into a clean jar.

Another method is to place 1 ounce dry herb in a clean, regular mouth jar with 2-3 tablespoons vodka or Everclear, just enough to moisten the herb so it will hold together in your hand when you squeeze it. Top with an Oster blender bottom, complete with rubber ring and blade. Holding the jar (so it doesn't spin off), chop the herb until somewhat fine. Let sit for about 12 hours. Add 7-9 ounces of good quality oil and top with blender bottom and blade. Hold onto the jar again so it doesn't spin off and blend on high for 3-5 minutes, until the mixture feels warm. Do this 5 times over the next 48 hours. If it is cold in your kitchen you may want to place your oil in a warm (not hot) water bath overnight. Strain the herb from the oil, using muslin, wringing out as much of the oil as you can. Store in a dark cool place. Will last up to 2 years if stored properly.

Herbs for When You Don't Feel Good

Now let's move on to individual herbs and their properties, healing uses and maybe a recipe or two to try.

We grow or have grown each of the herbs in this section and use them frequently. Please remember that we have no special expertise and did research that you can easily do for yourself. The library, websites, personal books, and local expertise were the source of our information.

Teas are common preparations for many herbs. They are easily produced and are mostly very enjoyable. Let them steep longer (10-15 minutes) to release more of the medicinal properties.

Poultices, salves, ointments, oils, and waters all have their place in the home first aid kit. The list of herbs and the information that follows is a collection that we have developed over several years. It briefly covers all the herbs we could find that had some valid research behind them and that we have grown either at the Georgeson Botanical Garden or our homes.

Anise Hyssop
(Agastache foeniculun)

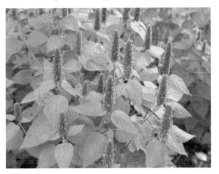

Anise hyssop is a perennial herb in less extreme climates. In Fairbanks, it is propagated by seed whether from reseeding itself or a seed package from a commercial grower. Our local nurseries sometimes have starter plants. The plant will grow to about 18-24 inches tall. It has a very sweet licorice flavor.

Medicinal Uses: Anise Hyssop is said to relieve the congestion of the common cold. It is used to strengthen the heart. It is diaphoretic (causes sweating) to reduce fever. The essential oil has shown to have antiviral properties to Herpes simplex 1 and 2. It is an aromatic digestant and prevents gas and bloating. It has sedative properties and is relaxing. Since it is antibacterial and anti-inflammatory it can be used in a salve or ointment to treat wounds. It is frequently prescribed in combination with other herbs for respiratory infections and bronchitis. Placing leaves in a very warm bath may relieve the itching of some rashes.

Parts used: leaves and flowers. Used in teas and salves.

Anise Hyssop medicinal tea: Place 1 tsp of dried anise hyssop in a tea ball or tea strainer. Put the tea ball in a cup. Pour very hot, boiling point, water over the tea and steep for 10 minutes. Remove the tea ball, put your feet up and enjoy.

Arnica

(Arnica Chamissonis, Arnica Montana)

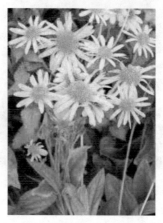

Arnica is perennial for us in Fairbanks. It is a low growing rather loose rosette or open growth in my garden that tends to flop along the ground. It is easy to start from seed and is available, occasionally, at nurseries or plant sales. It needs a slightly acidic soil and will not tolerate limed soil. It can grow from 1 to 2 feet tall when upright. Prefers full sun but will tolerate shade. Seeds can take from a month to 2 years to germinate. Germinates at about 55°F. Spreads by self-seeding and roots.

Parts used: flowers. Used in oils, liniments, and salves.

Medicinal Uses: A strong anti-inflammatory, liniments or oils infused with dried arnica flowers are an effective topical treatment for blunt force injury, strains, or sprains. Since ancient times arnica has been combined with calendula and St. John's Wort to relieve pain, fight infection and speed healing. Arnica should only be applied topically. Only a very small homeopathic dose is considered safe to take internally. Scientific studies are few and far between, but some have shown that arnica does reduce swelling and soreness from injury and seems to relieve acne. Gels and oils have, in some studies, been shown to relieve osteoarthritis. All species of arnica appear to have similar medical actions.

47

Arnica Infused Oil

Hot Method: Place a ratio of 1 part arnica leaf and/or flowers to 5 parts oil into a slow cooker or other low heat appliance. Heat on very low (110 to 115 degrees) for 4 hours. Cool, strain and pour into a sterile jar with an airtight lid. Keeps up to 1 year. This method produces a weaker strength than the cold method, but both are effective.

Cold Method: Place 1 part herb in sterile jar with 5-7 parts good oil. Cover with airtight lid and place in a cool, dark spot for 2-4 weeks. Shake every few days. Strain to remove herb, squeezing to get all the constituents you can. Pour into clean sterile jar. Keeps for up to 1 year. You can add 1 teaspoon citric acid or a few drops of rosemary essential oil to support shelf life.

Ashwagandha

(Withania somnifera)

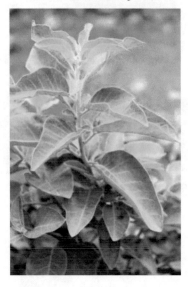

Ashwagandha is an annual in colder climates. It needs a warm place to grow. Sow seeds in flats or pots 10-12 weeks prior to frost-free days. Transplant into a sunny location, in well-drained soil. It prefers dry soil rather than wet after it is established.

Medicinal uses: Adaptogen, anti-inflammatory, antioxidant, good for immune system, fatigue, emaciation, degenerative disease, anxiety, asthma, arthritis, fibromyalgia and insulin resistance. Can improve memory.

Parts used: Mainly root, leaf, and berries. Used as decoction, a powder in food or as a tincture.

(Do not take with barbiturates or during pregnancy.)

Basil

(Ocimum basilicum)

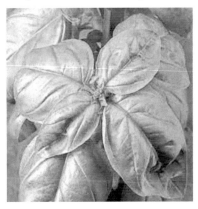

Basil is an annual herb with around 150 different species, grown in warmer regions of the world. It can be started from seed or from cuttings. It likes full sun or greenhouse and rich, moist, well-drained soil. Does well in warm garden spots or in pots. Start harvesting the top parts of the plant and some side leaves when the plant reaches 6-8 inches, snipping at the leaf junctions. Basil really starts growing when the temperature gets up to the 80s. The size of the plant is dependent on the variety and can be anywhere from 8 inches tall to 32 inches tall. There are as many flavors of basil as there are varieties. Young plants are found in all our nurseries, and many nurseries carry several varieties. They do like to be fed with a liquid fertilizer every two weeks.

Medicinal Uses: All varieties of basil share the compounds that can be helpful in treating or preventing acne, stress, pink eye, gout, heart attack, gastric upsets, pain, and wound healing. They also have strong antibacterial properties. Lab studies in India have shown that basil has "the potential to block or suppress" liver, stomach, and lung cancer. Basil can be used as basil water or tea for indigestion in addition to regular use as a seasoning herb. May also be made into a tincture. (Excessive supplementation of basil extracts may result in anti-fertility effects.)

Parts used: leaves

Basil Water: Place several leaves or 1 teaspoon of dried basil in the bottom of an 8-ounce glass. Muddle the fresh leaves a bit then cover with water. Allow to steep for 5 to 10 minutes. Drink after meals to prevent indigestion. This may have some sedative effect, so evening use is a plus.

Basil Pesto: Put 1 cup basil leaves, 2 tablespoons parmesan, 2 tablespoon pine nuts and 1-2 cloves garlic in blender or processor. Slowly add ¼ cup of olive oil as the machine runs. Process until creamy.

Blue Vervain

(Verbena hastata)

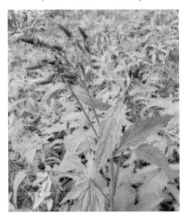

Blue Vervain is a native American plant that grows in disturbed sites and is commonly found in moist meadows, thickets, and pastures, as well as riversides, marshes, ditches, and river-bottom prairies of the lower US. Find a place in your garden that might be similar to these conditions. It is a perennial here in Fairbanks but not as prolific as in warmer areas. The seeds need to be stratified before sowing, by storing in a sealed, labeled container with wet sand or peat moss at 38-40 degrees F for three months. Then the seeds need light to germinate. Keep moist. Succeeds in any moderately fertile, well-drained but moisture-retentive soil in a sunny location. Sow seeds in early spring or transplant by root division in the spring. Basal cuttings can be taken in early summer. The shoots, with plenty of underground stem, can be used for transplanting. Self-seeds and spreads through rhizomes.

Parts used: Roots and leaves. For stronger remedies, pick before plant flowers and dry right away. Use as tea and poultice.

Medicinal uses: Blue Vervain relaxes the nervous system. Offers pain relief as a poultice. As tea, helps with headache, bladder discomfort and sore throat. Is a good expectorant. It also supports detoxification and stimulates digestion.

Caution: Blue vervain can interfere with blood pressure medication and hormone therapy. Large doses will induce vomiting and diarrhea.

Borage

(Borago officinalis)

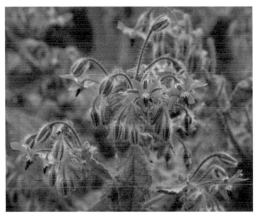

Borage is a perennial that can take over a garden spot it likes. It likes well drained soil in a medium pH range. Seeds can be sown directly in the garden after the last frost date. Plant ¼" to ½" deep, in rows 12 inches apart. Thin to at least 1 foot when the plants measure 4-6 inches tall. Self-seeds. The flowers have a pleasant cucumber-like flavor and add color and interest to salads.

Parts used: Leaves and flowers. Used as decoction, tea or poultice.

Medicinal uses: As a decoction, a cup or two a day can help enhance endorphins (feel good chemicals) in the brain. Tea helps with fever and a poultice helps with inflammation or swelling.

Catnip or Cat mint

(Nepeta Cataria)

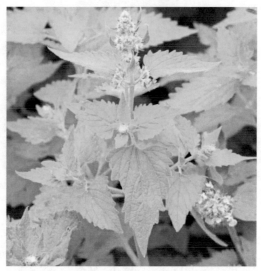

A member of the mint family and as such, can spread easily. Start seeds indoors and transplant into a sunny, well-drained location after last frost. Can be harvested throughout the season. Can be a perennial in some spots in Fairbanks.

Parts used: Leaves and flowering tops. Used as tea, poultice, or oil.

Medicinal uses: Promotes relaxation in humans. Catnip tea is a valuable drink for fever, because of its action in inducing sleep and producing perspiration without increasing the heat of the system. It is good in restlessness, colic, and nervousness, and is used as a mild nervine for children. Poultice for skin irritations. Oil can be used for mosquito repellant.

Chamomile

(Matericaria recutia)-German Chamomile
(Anthemis nobilis)-Roman Chamomile

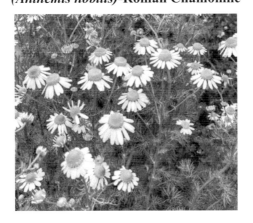

Chamomile has been used as a healing herb since the time of the Greek and Roman empires. Roman chamomile is a low growing perennial plant that is frequently used as a ground cover in more temperate climates. German chamomile is an annual herb that grows to about ½ to 1 feet tall. Both have white daisy-like flowers. It is rarely seen in nurseries or plant sales as it seeds or reseeds readily. Harvest flowers when in full bloom. Can harvest more than once a summer.

Parts used: Flowers. Used as tea, tincture, oil, salve and poultice.

Medicinal Uses: Roman chamomile (Anthemis nobilis) is used as an aromatic, bitter tonic, and stomach treatment. It makes a bitter tea. German chamomile (Matricaria recutia) is sweeter and has larger flowers. Both have anti-inflammatory, anti-bacterial, muscle relaxant, anti-spasmodic, anti-allergenic and sedative properties according to recent and ongoing research studies. The tea is used for lumbago (low back pain), rheumatic problems, and rashes as well as a sleep aid. Vapors are used for colds and asthma relief. Chamomile seems to be effective in reducing the nausea associated with pregnancy. It can be used as a poultice for skin rashes, skin problems, sunburn, burns, or irritated eyes.

Chamomile Tea: Place 1 teaspoon of dried chamomile flowers in a tea bag or tea strainer in a cup. Pour very hot water over flowers and steep for about 10 minutes. Remove flowers, relax, and enjoy.

Chamomile oil: 1 ounce dried flowers, powdered in a blender. Mix in 2 tablespoons vodka or enough to barely moisten the chamomile and let sit overnight. Add 7 ounces good quality oil and place in a water bath in a multi-cooker or slow-cooker. Use low heat (yogurt setting or lowest setting). Keep warm 3 hours or up to 3 days. You can also blend 3-5 minutes or until warm 5 times over 48 hours. Strain oil and bottle. Store in a cool dark place.

Chickweed

(Stellaria media)

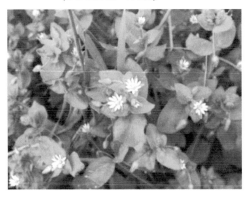

Chickweed is usually considered a scourge in our gardens and lawns. However, it is a nutrient powerhouse. It is a low growing annual plant in the carnation family. It has opposing oval leaves and small 5 petal flowers. The plant flowers and sets seed at the same time and spreads profusely.

Parts used: Leaves and flowers. Used as tea, tincture, and salve.

Medicinal Uses: Chickweed infusions have been used to treat bronchitis, pleurisy, gastritis, asthma, and sore throat because of its reportedly "unsurpassed" ability to cool fevers and fight infections. Chickweed's diuretic action helps eliminate toxins from the system and reduces retention of fluids. Fresh chickweed is effective as a poultice for drawing out splinters, insect stingers, for minor burns and to dissolve warts or treat boils. It may also relieve rheumatic pain. It's vulnerary (wound healing) action will reduce healing time on cuts and other skin abrasions. It also has emollient qualities and will soothe itching and irritation of eczema or psoriasis.

An infusion may be added to a bath for relief of inflamed skin. It provides relief to swollen and painful hemorrhoids. It is an excellent source of vitamins A, D, B complex, C, rutin, (an accompanying flavonoid) as well as iron, calcium, potassium, phosphorus, zinc, manganese, sodium, copper, and silica. Chickweed can be used as an infusion, tincture, or tea. Fresh leaves or flowers can be added to salads. It is generally considered safe for all external applications and comsuption. There has been 1 report of toxicity after ingestion of a large amount of the infused herb, however, there are no other documented reports of toxicity.

Chickweed Poultice: Chop fresh chickweed leaves and stems in sufficient quantity to cover the area being treated. Sprinkle the herb with water and place over the area. Cover the herbal mass with a strip of wet gauze to hold it in place. You can simmer older, tougher plants in a small amount of water of a 50/50 mixture of vinegar and water for about 5 minutes and then apply to skin when mixture is cold.

Cilantro, Coriander

(Coriandrum sativum)

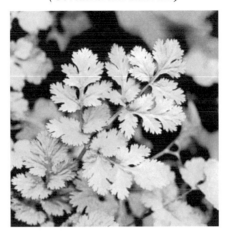

Cilantro is one of the world's oldest herbs. The seeds are known as coriander. Direct sow outdoors after last frost or start seeds in propagation starter cubes or plugs indoors, six weeks before planting outdoors, being careful not to disturb the root ball as it will cause bolting. Will grow in a relatively wide pH range between 6.1 (mildly acidic) and 7.8 (mildly alkaline), with an ideal range between 6.5 and 7.5. Plant 9-12 inches apart. For seeds, plant in direct sun. For leaves, plant in partial shade. Prefers a deep, fertile soil which can be either light or heavy, as long as it is well drained. It does prefer cooler temperatures.

Parts used: Leaves, stems and green seeds. Eat fresh or use as tincture.

Medicinal uses: Promotes the flow of bile. Helps mobilize heavy metals including mercury, cadmium, lead, and aluminum from bones, teeth, central nervous system and other body tissues. Combine tincture with tincture of dandelion or red clover (50:50) to dispel toxins through the urine. It can lower your cholesterol and can help with digestion. It is rich in Vitamins A, C, and K and several minerals, such as calcium potassium, iron, magnesium, and manganese. The seeds have been used to treat indigestion, nausea, and dysentery.

Comfrey

(Symphytum officinale)

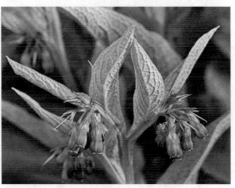

Comfrey is usually a perennial herb in Fairbanks. Grows well in partial shade, in well -drained soil. Can be grown from seed but is easier to cultivate from root cuttings, which should be planted horizontally about 3 inches deep and 24 inches apart. Any cut root will sprout a new plant. Leaves make a great compost activator. It can be 5 feet tall and a yard wide in warmer climates, but is generally much smaller in Fairbanks.

Parts used: Leaves and roots. Used as oil and salve.

Medicinal Uses: Disclaimer: Comfrey may be toxic to the liver in both humans and animals and caution should be taken if used internally. Comfrey has been used as a bone mender and healer of wounds for centuries. It is often used as a poultice but is also effective when added to salves, ointments, tinctures and decoctions for inflammation, sprained ankles, eczema, swellings, bruises, cuts, scrapes, insect bites, and burns. Studies have found it effective in the treatment of dermatitis, viral skin infections and lower leg ulcers. The crushed fresh leaf placed on a rash or poison ivy blister will bring relief.

Salve: Heat 2 cups olive oil with 2 tablespoons of dried comfrey leaf, 2 tablespoons lavender flowers, and 2 tablespoons calendula flowers over very low heat in a double boiler or in a slow cooker. Stir often. Simmer for about 30 minutes up to 3 hours, but don't let it bubble in the middle. Strain into a clean, sterile bowl and discard herbs. Melt ½ cup beeswax pastilles or grated beeswax and add to herbal oil. Stir well and pour into sterile glass jars or tins. Label and date for safety.

Dandelion

(Araxacum officinale)

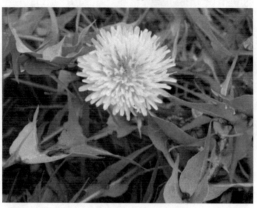

Dandelion is a pervasive flowering plant found throughout the world. Most consider it a weed, but it has many useful properties. It is one of very few plants that the root, leaf and flower are all used medicinally. It is a single-stemmed plant with a taproot and yellow flowers. It is native to Europe and Asia and was brought to North America as a food crop. A single plant can produce 5000 seeds which are then blown as far as 300 yards or more from the plant. It is a food source for some lepidoptera (butterflies and moths), caterpillars and although not a highly nutritious food for bees, they do feed on the pollen. It has culinary uses: leaves as a vegetable, flowers as wine and the root as a coffee substitute. When harvesting the roots, leave a couple to grow more.

Parts used: Roots, leaves, and flowers. Used for tea and tincture.

Medicinally Uses: Dandelion is used for digestive issues, joint pain, and urinary tract problems, constipation, as well as liver and bile issues. It is anti-inflammatory, anti-carcinogenic, and anti-oxidative. It has amazing detoxification properties for liver and is a good blood tonic. The bitter resina and potent oils stimulate the liver into a positive loop that promotes proper digestion. The root and leaves are rich in antioxidants such as vitamin C and luteolin, which prevent free radical damage. Dandelions are a good source of calcium, vitamin A and probably the richest source of vitamin K, all of which are good for bones. The phyto-nutrients and essential fatty acids reduce inflammation in the body. Recent studies have found that dandelion root extract is effective against several kinds of cancer cells in lab tests. Human trials of all herbs are very limited in this country. It has been suggested that dandelion leaves, which are rich in choline, may aid in restoring memory. Since dandelion leaves are diuretic, the water loss can result in weight loss and lowered blood pressure. You can consume any part of the plant in a salad, as a vegetable, a smoothie, or a tea. Each part of the plant contains alkaloids, steroids, and triterpenoids that have healthful effects on the body.

Dandelion Flower Tea: Wash 3 to 5 dandelion flowers in a colander under cold running water to remove dirt and bugs. Remove the yellow petals. Use other parts of the plant in different ways or compost. Put the petals in a quart glass jar and cover with 2 cups boiling water. Add stevia leaves or other sweetener to taste. Steep for 5 minutes until color and flavor are infused in the water. Add 2 tablespoons lime juice, stir well and strain. Serve hot or iced. Makes about 2 cups.

Dill

(Anetheum graveolens)

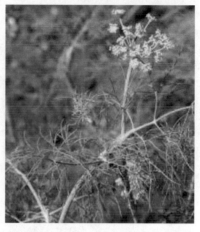

Dill has many culinary uses. It germinates quickly. You can direct seed it in your garden after last frost or you can start indoors and transplant to sandy, well-drained soil. Space 10 inches apart.

Parts used: Seeds and leaves. Seeds for medicinal applications (tea and decoctions) Leaves for culinary.

Medicinal uses: Chewing dill seeds freshens bad breath. A daily cup of strong tea (1 tbsp. dill seed simmered 15 min in 1 pint water) may help reduce risk of breast cancer.

Echinacea

(Echinacea angustifolia)

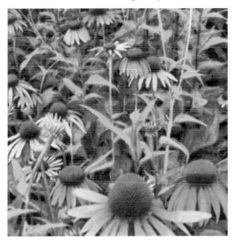

Also known as coneflowers, they are not fussy and will endure most conditions. However, give them rich, well-drained soil and plenty of sunshine and plants will thrive. Generous amounts of organic compost or aged animal manure mixed into the ground prior to planting will vastly improve the health of plants. Will tolerate heat and drought. Grow from direct-seeding, nursery stock or division. Best started indoors with cold stratification of the seeds. Takes 10-20 days to germinate. They are perennials in many parts of the country but not here in Fairbanks. 90-120 days from seed to flower. Bees and birds love the flowers.

Parts used: Flowers and (3-year-old) mature roots. Used as tea, tinctures, poultices. Flowers are less effective than roots.

Medicinal uses: Immune system booster! Increases the production of white killer cells in the body to help eliminate infectious diseases, especially the common cold, the flu, and other upper respiratory infections. Best used at very early onset of symptoms. Also used against many other infections, especially combined with other herbs. Using it "just in case" will negate its immune-stimulating properties. Use judiciously as needed.

Caution: May cause dry mouth, digestive upsets and rashes. Not advised to use if you have an autoimmune disease.

Fennel

(Foeniculum vulgare)

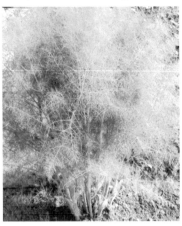

Grow in full sun, in well-drained soil. Stake. Sow about 12 inches apart, covering with ¼-inches soil. Harvest when seeds turn brown. Cover umbels with cheesecloth as seeds ripen to catch them.

Parts used: Seeds. Used as tea and decoction.

Medicinal uses: Helps relieve bloating, gas, and abdominal cramps. Has estrogenic properties that help ease menopause and menstrual symptoms.

Caution: Avoid fennel essential oil if pregnant or breastfeeding.

Feverfew

(Tanacetu parthenium)

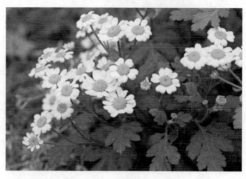

Native to the Balkan Peninsula, feverfew is now found in Australia, Europe, China, Japan, and North Africa. In the mid-19th century, feverfew was introduced in the United States. The plant grows along roadsides, fields, waste areas, and along the borders of woods from eastern Canada to Maryland and westward to Missouri. Feverfew was also known as "medieval aspirin" or the "aspirin" of the 18th century. It has been planted around houses to purify the air because of its strong, lasting odor, and a tincture of its blossoms can be used as an insect repellant. Sow in a sunny spot in spring or early summer. A self-seeder so leave a few plants when harvesting to seed for the next year. Do not confuse with tansy (tanacetu vulgare). Tansy has no medicinal effects.

Parts used: Leaves. Used as tea and tincture.

Medicinal uses: Has a mild tranquilizing effect that helps ease the tension that leads to headaches. Traditionally used for the treatment of fevers, migraine headaches, rheumatoid arthritis, stomach aches, toothaches, insect bites, worms, infertility, reduce inflammation, boost respiratory health and problems with menstruation and labor during childbirth.

Caution: Fresh feverfew leaves can cause mouth ulcers. Do not use during pregnancy (can cause bleeding) or if allergic to ragweed.

Horseradish

(Armoracia rusticana)

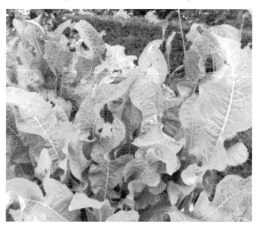

Horseradish is a plant that has been used for the last 3,000 years. Both root and leaves were used as medicine in the Middle Ages. It has been used as a condiment for meat easily since the 18th century and probably before. Grows easily in most climates. Grow in a contained spot because it has a habit of taking over. Roots can be harvested any time after the leaves appear.

Parts used: Root. Use fresh, in vinegar tinctures, to make salves and tea.

Medicinal uses: Can clear blocked sinuses, loosen chest congestion, and promotes circulation. It is a useful diuretic. May also help ease urinary tract infections. Has many antioxidants. It has been used as a treatment for rheumatism and to help prevent inflammation, whether from injury or arthritis. Native Americans used it to stimulate the glands, stave off scurvy and as a treatment for the common cold, especially as an expectorant. May also help prevent different forms of cancer. Can stimulate digestion and bowel movements. Stimulates bile production in the gallbladder, thus also aiding digestion. Rubbing the fresh root on skin discolorations (melasma), one to several times a week may help them fade.

Caution: Small children (under 4), pregnant or breastfeeding women should avoid. Horseradish may aggravate intestinal ulcers or inflammatory bowel disease. Could be a concern for people with kidney disorders since it might increase urine flow. Also do not use if you have low thyroid function or if you take thyroxine.

Fire Cider Tonic-Basic Recipe: Place 2 large onions, rough chopped; 2 heads garlic, rough chopped, skins on; two 3-4 inch pieces fresh ginger, rough chopped, peel on; ½ cup grated horseradish; 1 tsp. cayenne pepper; raw apple cider vinegar to cover. Place all ingredients in a 2-quart jar and cover completely with vinegar, leaving 1-2 inches of headspace. Screw a non-corrosive lid on the jar and place in a warm place, out of direct sunlight. Shake the jar every day for 4 weeks. Strain out the solids and decant the liquid into a clean jar. Refrigerate the tonic for up to a year. You can add different herbs that work best for you. To be taken at the first onset of a cold or flu. 1-2 ounces straight or mix with warm water and a touch of honey.

Horsetail

(Equisetum arvense)

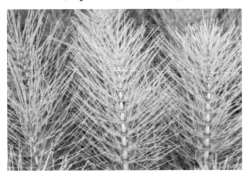

The ancient Romans used horsetail medicinally. The ancient Greeks used it for wound healing, a diuretic, and a styptic (something to stop blood flow). It grows easily and is considered a weed. Propagates by active spores. Enjoys shady, moist areas.

Parts used: Aerial parts, especially when they reach up rather than droop down. (Down drooping contains oxalate crystals.) Used for tea, tinctures, poultices, salves, and powdered.

Medicinal uses: Rich in silica that can help our bodies form collagen, it can be important for tissue, skin, bone, cartilage, and ligaments. Helps promote healthy skin and nails. Helps mend broken bones, treat, and prevent osteoporosis. Promotes urination and is a remedy for bladder and urinary-tract infections. Strengthens bladder wall, helps heal stomach ulcers and remove kidney stones. Strengthens hair shafts when used as a rinse. High also in calcium, magnesium, and sulfur.

Caution: Long-term use not recommended. May deplete body of thiamin (B1), although tincturing or decocting can help remedy this. Do not use horsetail if you have edema, gout, heart problems or kidney inflammation. Another species E. Palustre is poisonous to horses and is recommended not to ingest. The juice or sap of these plants contains tiny oxalate crystals that are shaped like tiny needles. Chewing on these plants can cause immediate pain and irritation to the lips, mouth, and tongue. In severe cases, they may cause breathing problems by causing swelling in the mouth and throat.

Lavender

(Lavandula spp)

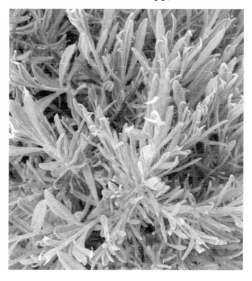

Lavender is another of those perennial herbs that we can grow pretty successfully as annuals, in interior Alaska. They prefer well drained, even slightly dry soil and direct sun but will manage with some afternoon shade. Lavender loves to be warm. The plant grows to about 18 high in my garden. Most years it blooms. Plants of many varieties are available at our greenhouses. Hidcote and Munstead are the hardiest of the bunch.

Parts used: Flowers and leaves. Used as teas, tinctures, oils, and salves.

Medicinal Uses: Lavender is most often used for restlessness, insomnia, nervousness, and depression. In lab studies, lavender provided as much improvement in mood as pharmaceuticals. Lavender is also commonly used to treat stomach issues, such as flatulence, loss of appetite, vomiting and nausea. Inhaling lavender aromas relieves migraine headaches in some people. It relaxes muscles when massaged into skin and has healing and soothing effects on rashes, burns, bug bites and other skin problems. Also good for bacterial and fungal infections and wounds. Lavender seems to have a sedative effect when taken as a tea. Reduces tension, anxiety, and depression. Lavender flower tea is good for colic. Lavender tincture is good for suppressing coughs.

Lavender Tea: Crush 2 teaspoons to 2 tablespoons lavender flowers and or leaves. Put in a cup or teapot. Add hot water to fill the cup or pot. Steep until it cools. Drink the cooled tea and enjoy the relaxing aroma. Chamomile may be added to enhance the relaxing effect.

Lavender oil: 1 ounce dried lavender flowers, powdered. You can do this in a blender**. Add 2 tablespoons vodka (100 proof is best) and pulse. Let set overnight. Next day, add 7 ounces oil and blend for 3-5 minutes until it becomes warm. Do this about 5 times over the next 48 hours. Strain into a clean jar. Great for headaches and sunburns.

**A regular Oster blender bottom fits on a regular mouth jar. Use a jar instead of the blender pitcher. Hold the jar as you blend because sometimes it can spin off. What a mess!

Lemongrass

(Cymbopogon citratus)

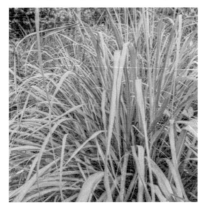

Lemongrass is a warm or temperate climate native herb. We are all used to it in Asian cuisine. The plant is propagated by root cuttings or division. It grows to about 3 feet tall with slender long leaves. It is treated as an annual here although it is perennial in more moderate climates. It is easy to grow in pots in a warm place and loves composted soil. You can also apply a liquid fertilizer every couple of weeks to encourage growth. It starts slow but grows quickly as the weather warms. Needs to be watered regularly.

Parts used: leaves

Medicinal Uses: Lemongrass is commonly used to treat stomach upsets, digestive tract spasms, and coughs. It has some anti-bacterial and anti-fungal properties that bear further research. It is used to treat high blood pressure, convulsions, muscle pain and abdominal pain. It may have the ability to reduce fever, stimulate the uterus, and it has antioxidant and anti-inflammatory properties. These uses and its effectiveness are being confirmed by research as well as its apparent ability to kill cancer cells in the lab. Lemongrass oils are used in aromatherapy, insect repellents or mixed with other herb oils to treat many conditions. The tea is used for the treatment of the common cold or coughs.

Medicinal Tea: Place 10-12 lemongrass leaves in 2 cups of boiling water. Add one generous slice of ginger and honey to taste. Steep 10 minutes. Strain and drink 1 cup every 8 hours for colds, stomach aches, flu, or headaches. May be used as either a hot or cold beverage.

Lemon Balm
(Melissa officinalis)

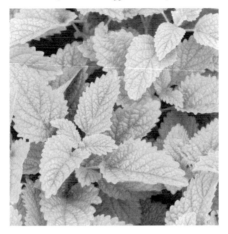

Grows freely in any soil and can be propagated by seeds, cuttings, or division of roots in spring or autumn. The roots may be divided into small pieces, with three or four buds to each, and planted 2 feet apart in ordinary garden soil. Weed and cut off the decayed stalks in autumn, and then stir the ground between the roots. Lemon Balm is most often an annual in Fairbanks.

Parts used: leaves for tea, infused oil, balm and tincture.

Medicinal uses: Considered a calming herb. It was used as far back as the Middle Ages to reduce stress and anxiety, promote sleep, improve appetite, and ease pain and discomfort from indigestion (including gas and bloating, as well as colic). Also good for menstrual cramps and PMS. Has been used for herpes and its astringent and antibacterial qualities have skin care applications, not only as a lip balm, but also as a facial cleanser and moisturizer.

Lemon Verbena

(Lippia citriodora)

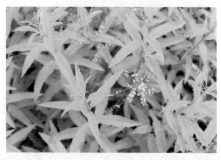

One of our favorite herbs for tea, lemon verbena is best purchased and grown in a warm place, a sunny deck or greenhouse. Grows well in pots. Fertilize regularly and water when the top 2 inches of soil are dry.

Parts used: Leaves. Used as tea or decoction.

Medicinal uses: As a decoction, has sedative actions, helps with fever. Also good for indigestion and flatulence. Stimulates skin and stomach. Helps stop muscle spasms. Reduces oxidative stress levels in the body.

Caution: Could worsen kidney disease. Some people suffer a mild dermatitis allergic response.

Marjoram

(Origanum majorana)

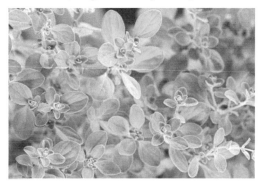

Marjoram is a member of the mint family and has been grown in the Mediterranean, Northern Africa and Western Asia for thousands of years. When growing marjoram plants, it's generally best to start the seeds indoors during late winter or early spring. Push seeds just below the soil surface. Seedlings can be transplanted outdoors once all threat of frost has passed. Marjoram should be located in areas receiving full sun with light, well-drained soil. Will grow in a relatively wide pH range between 6.1 (mildly acidic) and 8.5 (alkaline) with a preferred range between 6.5 and 7.5 and should be spaced between 15 and 18 inches (38 - 45 cm) apart.

Parts used: Leaves, mostly for tea.

Medicinal uses: Marjoram is commonly used for coughs, runny nose, common colds, menstrual pain, and digestive problems. It can be used as a tea or extract, fresh or dry. It also has antioxidant and anti-inflammatory properties. Good for nausea, flatulence, stomach cramps, diarrhea or constipation, a cup or two of tea can help alleviate symptoms. A traditional medicine to restore hormonal balance and regulate the menstrual cycle. Whether you're dealing with the unwanted monthly symptoms of PMS or menopause, this herb can provide relief for women of all ages. Considered an emmenagogue, which means it can be used to help start menstruation. It's also been used traditionally by

80

nursing moms to promote breast milk production. Can also help manage blood sugar.

Mullein

(Verbascum thapsus)

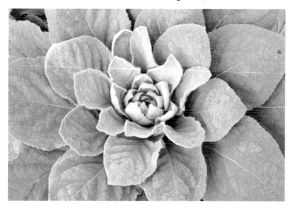

Mullein is a wooly looking plant that grows bigger in warmer climates than in Fairbanks. Seeds need light to germinate. Pat them onto the soil but don't cover. Transplant after first leaves appear. Spike with flowers appear the second year but you can harvest the leaves the first year. Harvest flowers, leaves, and buds the second year, leaving some to self-seed.

Parts used: Leaves and flowers. Used as tea, poultice or infused oil.

Medicinal uses: Great for coughs, earaches, and sore throats. Good for asthma. Analgesic, expectorant, and anti-bacterial. It is also a demulcent that creates a soothing anti-inflammatory coating over mucous membranes in the lungs, throat, and bronchial passages. A fresh poultice is a good first aid treatment for minor wounds, burns and insect bites. Seems to have some strong antiviral effects. A test tube study found it to be useful against the influenza virus. Other studies have suggested it might be useful in fighting a strain of herpes virus. Lab tests in 2002 found that mullein helped kill certain types of bacteria, including *Staphylococcus aureus.*

Caution: Seeds are considered toxic, use only flowers or leaves. Some people may get contact dermatitis from handling the leaves.

Mullein Tea: Use 1-2 teaspoons of dry, loose leaf in 1 cup boiled water. Let steep 10-15 minutes. Can drink 3-4 cups a day.

Nettle

(Urtica dioica)

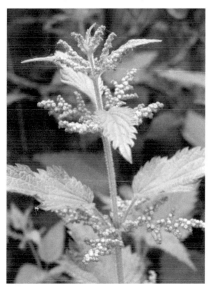

Stinging Nettle is a perennial herb growing nearly worldwide. It occurs in moist sites along streams, meadow, and ditches, on mountain slopes, in woodland clearings, and in disturbed areas. Stinging nettle generally grows in deep, rich, moist soil and doesn't do well in areas of drought. It reproduces by rhizomes and seeds and can form dense colonies covering an acre or more. It is considered a noxious weed in some areas.

Parts used: leaves and roots. Used in teas, decoctions, dry powder, tinctures, and salves.

Medicinal uses: High in vitamin K1, vitamin C, folate, and beta-carotene (vitamin A), calcium, iron, and silica. Leaves and roots are diuretics, good for urinary tract infections, and kidney stones. A blood purifier. Helpful for congestion, allergies, joint and muscle pain, circulation, hair loss, urinary infections, nose bleeds, eczema, PMS, menopause, and fatigue. According to a study published in the Journal of Ethnopharmacology, stinging nettle has components that contain natural anesthetic and anti-inflammatory compounds. The tiny hairs that cover the nettle leaves contain histamine, serotonin, and other chemicals that help to lessen pain by stimulating pain neurons. You can enjoy this benefit by either steeping it in hot water or applying it directly to the skin around the painful area.

Caution: Fresh leaves have stinging hairs that can cause rashes. Only young leaves should be eaten because older leaves develop gritty particles called cystoliths which can act as an irritant to the kidneys.

Oregano

(Origanum vulgare)

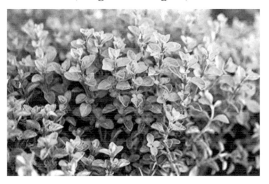

Oregano is another Mediterranean herb that is popular all over the world. It is a perennial in warm places but for us Northern folks, it is an annual. Originally grown in Greece, the name means "mountain joy". It loves the sun, so ensure that your placement has full, strong sun for strong flavor. It is easily grown in Fairbanks and all the nurseries will have a variety or two. You can start it from seed but can also use cuttings from an established plant. Start 6-10 weeks before first frost or plant the seeds/cuttings in well-drained soil any time after the last spring frost. The soil should be around 70ºF. Plant 8 to 10 inches apart. The plant usually grows no more than a foot high with a mounding growth habit. It makes a nice edging plant for a bed. Allow oregano plants to grow to about 4 inches tall and then pinch or trim lightly to encourage a denser and bushier plant. Regular trimming will not only cause the plant to branch again, but also avoid legginess. Oregano doesn't need quite as much water as most herbs. As the amount of watering depends on many variables, just water when the soil feels dry to the touch. Remember that it's better to water thoroughly and less often. If you have a container, water until the water comes out of the drainage holes in the bottom of the container.

Parts used: Leaves and flowers. Used as tea, tincture, and oil.

Medicinal Uses: Oregano is antioxidant, antiseptic, preservative, antibacterial, antiviral, and antifungal. It has been shown to be effective against chronic candidiasis using enteric coated capsules. It is also used to treat yeast infections and other infections. Its anti-microbial properties are probably due to the thymol and carvacrol. Tea or tincture can be taken for viral or bacterial colds and upper respiratory infections. Strong medicine for many infections. Oregano has been used in the treatment of several ailments such as diarrhea, stomach upset and nausea. The essential oil is used to treat skin problems when diluted 50% or more with a carrier oil. Use the oil for athlete's foot or other fungal infections. It is commonly administered as a medicinal tea for gastric upsets. It has also been used to treat myriad problems from asthma to Rheumatoid Arthritis but there are no lab results or research to support that at the present.

Oregano Tea: Place 1 to 2 teaspoons of dried or fresh oregano in a cup. Pour boiling water over the leaves and steep for 10 minutes.

Parsley

(Petroselinum crispum, Curly)
(Petroselinum Neapolitanum, Flat-leaf)

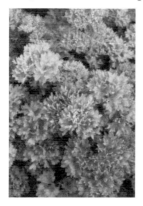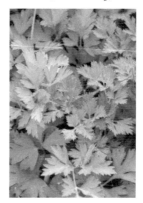

Parsley is native to the Mediterranean. Throughout time parsley was believed to have many unusual and magical uses. For example, it was once believed that this herb was evil and if you are in love, you should never cut parsley, or it would cut short and ruin your love. For a head start in the garden, plant seeds in individual pots indoors 10 to 12 weeks before the last spring frost. For better germination, soak the seeds overnight. Use a fluorescent light to help the seedlings grow, make sure it remains at least two inches above the leaves at all times. Otherwise, plant 3 to 4 weeks before the last spring frost because parsley is a slow starter. (The plants can handle the cold weather.) It can take up to 3 weeks for the plants to sprout. Plant in moist, rich soil about 6 to 10 inches apart. To ensure the best growth, the soil should be around 70°F. When the leaf stems have three segments, parsley is ready to be harvested. Cut leaves from the outer portions of the plant whenever you need them. Leave the inner portions to mature.

Parts used: Leaves. Best used fresh in large amounts, as in pesto or salads.

Medicinal uses: High in vitamin K1, vitamin C, folate, and beta-carotene. Rich in antioxidants and nutrients that protect eyes (lutein and zeaxanthin). Leaves and roots are diuretics, good for urinary tract infections, kidney, stones, cystitis, and edema. (Roots are stronger than leaves.) Has been used for high blood pressure, allergies, and inflammatory diseases. Improves digestion, bloating and gas. Good for bad breath.

Caution: Avoid in large amounts during pregnancy and lactation or if on blood-thinning medications. Can cause photosensitivity rash in some. (rare)

Chimichurri Recipe: Blend 1 bunch flat leaf parsley, 8 cloves garlic, ¾ cups extra virgin olive oil, ¼ cup red wine vinegar, juice of ¼ lime or lemon, 1 tablespoon diced red onion, 1 teaspoon dried oregano, 1 teaspoon black pepper, ½ teaspoon salt in a blender or food processor until well blended. Serve on meats or as a dip with crackers.

Peppermint

(Mentha piperita)

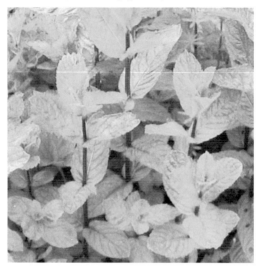

Ancient Egyptians, Romans and Greeks cultivated and used peppermint for indigestion and to sooth their stomachs. Peppermint is a hybrid cross between wild mint and spearmint. It is sterile and must be grown from cuttings or divisions. The seeds that you may see are seeds produced by parent plants fertilizing each other and producing seeds. It is almost always available at our greenhouses in the Spring. This is another perennial in zones 5 to 9 that we treat as an annual. This is a low growing plant that can become invasive if not regularly trimmed. Good as a container plant. It has spikes of lavender-pink flowers.

Parts used: The leaves are used to produce tea, oil, and tincture.

Medicinal Uses: Peppermint is used to treat the common cold, indigestion, nausea, stomachache, and menstrual disorders. The most prominent of the active ingredients is menthol, which is responsible for the burning, cooling sensation. Can help relieve itching. It calms coughs and strengthens the immune system. It has both anti-microbial and antioxidant qualities. Headaches, nerve pain, toothaches, general body aches and muscle pain seem to respond to external application of peppermint creams, oils, and salves. One study showed peppermint to be as effective at easing minor headaches as 1,000mg of acetaminophen. Peppermint oil, diluted with water can help rashes, acne, and dry skin due to infection, itchiness, and allergy. It is an excellent inhalant either from oils or candles to generate a heightened level of energy and focus.

Caution: Consumption or use of pure peppermint oil can irritate the digestive track or the skin so it should be diluted with either a carrier oil or water/alcohol. Although peppermint is good for digestion, it can aggravate heartburn. Discontinue if digestive problems worsen.

Peppermint Extract: Strip leaves from stems of peppermint until you have 1 cup. Place leaves in a sterile jar and crush or muddle to release the oil. Pour vodka, bourbon, or rum over the leaves until covered. Mash the leaves down with a spoon to make sure they are covered. Seal and let sit for 3 -4 weeks, shaking occasionally. Start tasting at 2 ½ weeks to find your perfect flavor. The longer it sits the stronger it gets. Strain when it reaches your preferred taste and bottle. Can be used in water as a gargle or digestive.

Plantain

(Plantago major)

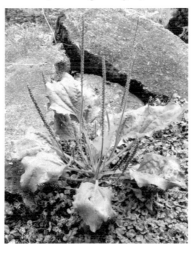

Plantain was considered to be one of the nine sacred herbs by the ancient Saxon people and has been celebrated in Anglo-Saxon poetry as the "mother of herbs." There are more than 200 species of plantain and nearly as many recorded uses for this humble herb. Plantain is native to northern and central Asia and Europe. Early colonists brought plantain to North America as one of their favored healing remedies. Native Americans called this persistent herb "white man's foot" as it is often found growing along well-trodden foot paths. The Latin generic name means "sole of the foot." The indigenous Americans adopted many of the traditional European uses for this beneficial herb. They also used the plant to draw out the poison of rattlesnake bite, to soothe rheumatic pain, as a poultice to treat battle wounds, and as an eyewash. They used the fresh young leaves and seeds in their diet. Plantain is a widespread weedy plant with a 6-to-25-inch flower stalk. It can be grown from seed. It is a self-seeding plant and can be found growing wild in most weedy areas. Prefers full sun to partial shade and will tolerate a wide range of soil conditions, including rocks and sand. It can be direct sown outdoors in mid-spring or started indoors in early spring and transplanted out in late spring.

Germination rates can be enhanced with a one-week period of cold stratification prior to sowing.

Parts used: Leaves. Used as tea, tincture, salve or poultice. Can also be used as a dry powder for a styptic.

Medicinal Uses: Plantain leaves contain mucilage tannins and salicylic acid. Traditionally used to relieve diarrhea, treat lung conditions, and similar conditions relating to excess bleeding and inflammation. Classified as a diuretic, alternative, astringent, and vulnerary. Also has antimicrobial, antihistamine, and anti-inflammatory benefits. It is used as a detox tea in Chinese traditional Medicine. It is popular as a cosmetic herb for sore or irritated skin. Crushed leaves in a decoction or juice may be used as a cooling tonic. Poultices using leaves are effective in healing wounds and preventing infection. Plantain leaves can be crushed and applied directly to a cut or scrape. It can be made into a decoction or tincture for coagulating blood. An ointment, salve or gel with plantain also has the ability to heal burns, wounds, insect bites, or bruises.

Salve: 1 cup fresh plantain leaves, 1 ½ cup olive oil or coconut oil, 1 Tbsp + 1 tsp packed grated beeswax, ½ to 1 tsp Tea Tree essential oil.

Clean, chop or grind leaves. Put in sterile glass jar and cover with oil. Put a cover on the jar to keep dust and bugs out. Let sit in a cool, dark place for 4 to 6 weeks. Strain. Melt the beeswax and add to the oil, stirring to combine. Stir in the Tea Tree essential oil and pour into containers.

Quick method: Place a folded towel in the bottom of a slow cooker. Put the jar of leaves and oil on the towel and add water up to the middle of the jar. Turn the cooker on the very lowest setting and keep warm for 12-24 hours. When oil is infused, strain. Melt beeswax in double boiler. Add oil and mix thoroughly. Cool slightly and add the Tea Tree essential oil or any other essential oil. Pour into sterile tin or jar. Use to heal skin abrasions and insect bites.

Raspberry

(Rubus idaeus, Rubus strigosus)

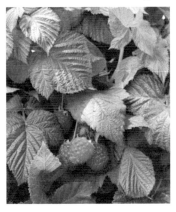

Wild raspberries can be found in disturbed soil, or on roadsides. Thrives in moisture-retentive, fertile, slightly acidic soils, which are well-drained and weed free. Dislikes soggy soils and shallow chalky soils. In the garden, for best results, plant in a sheltered, sunny place, although they will tolerate part shade. Bare-root canes in the garden or in containers, should be planted between April and October or when the soil is not frozen. Raspberries are usually planted in rows and trained along a post and wire system. But, if you have a smaller garden, you can still grow raspberries, either in containers, or train them up a single post. The flowers are self-fertile and pollinated by insects, so avoid a very windy site unless you can put up windbreaks or shelterbelts. Also, the fruiting side branches of some cultivars are very long and may break in the wind. Before planting, clear the site of perennial weeds, as these are difficult to control once raspberries are established. Space the plants around 18in–2ft apart, then add a 3 inches thick mulch of bulky organic matter. Avoid mushroom compost or overly rich farmyard manure, which can burn the new shoots.

Parts used: Leaves. Used as tea, decoction, or tincture.

Medicinal uses: Leaves are a remedy for cold and flu symptoms. Also used as tea for relieving menstrual discomfort and as a uterine tonic. Good during pregnancy.

Rhodiola

(Rhodiola rosea, Rhodiola Intefrifolia, T. crenulate)

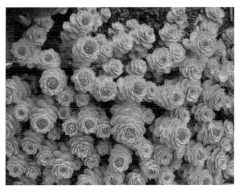

Rhodiola thrives in rocky, silty soil in northern and arctic climates. It grows wild in Alaska; however cultivated varieties are available. Remember if you forage, do not decimate wild stock. It is a small low growing plant (2-15 inches) with fleshy leaves. It is also called roseroot, golden root, Aaron's Rod, Arctic's Rod, and some other common names. Grows naturally where temperatures dip below freezing.

In cold climates, sow the seeds directly outside. Exposing the seeds to two or more months of winter weather, especially snow cover, triggers their germination. Takes 2-4 weeks to germinate, optimally at about 50°. You can start indoors by refrigerating seeds up to 6 weeks, then sprinkling on top of moist soil. Keep cool. Be especially careful of roots when transplanting. Each rhodiola plant has only one gender of flowers, either male or female. Plants require the help of bees or flies for pollination. If growing the plant for its roots, it takes four or five years to produce a sizable harvest. Russian rhodiola self-sows when growing in a favorable environment. It may be difficult to completely remove the plant from your garden.

Parts used: Mostly roots but leaves can be eaten. Used as tea, decoctions, and tinctures

96

Medicinal Uses: Rhodiola is an adaptogen which is a building and nourishing herb.   The few studies have been inconclusive.   It has traditionally been used to increase stamina, endurance, and strength in athletes.   Rhodiola is also used to treat various types of depression and anxiety.   Especially those associated with Seasonal Affective Disorder (SAD) in dark northern winters.   Studies seem to indicate a modulation of stress with the herb.   Rhodiola is an astringent and therefore is sometimes used to treat wounds, address diarrhea and control bleeding. Chinese Medicine uses rhodiola to treat heart and lung conditions as it is believed to move blood.   Benefits the nervous system and glandular systems. Can also be swabbed on gums or used as gargle for treating pyorrhea. Recent studies seem to show that rhodiola may be helpful in treating some cancers, such as colon and breast.   One study found that mouth sores were reduced in chemotherapy patients and improved white blood cell counts. Nearly all the information on rhodiola is speculation based on traditional uses and beliefs, not from scientifically controlled studies.

Rhodiola Tincture: Use 1 part rhodiola root to 2 parts vodka in a sterile jar. Cover with a tight-fitting lid and shake well. Put it in a dark, cool place and let it sit for 6 to 8 weeks. If the root swells above the vodka, add a little more to keep the root covered.   Strain through cheesecloth or muslin and squeeze to get every bit of the constituents of the herb.   Recommended dosage is 2-4 ml a day. Commercial rhodiola products may not be pure and may have other fillers added.

Rose

(Rosa spp, R. alba, R. damascene, R.centifolia)

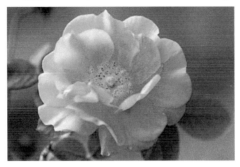

Roses are difficult to grow in Interior Alaska unless you are careful to get rugosa stock or some of the newer Canadian developments. I am a rose addict and have some in ground that vary from 2 feet tall and 2 feet wide to 5 foot tall and 4 feet wide. Various greenhouses have both roses for in ground and those lovely hybrids for a season. I have a limited success wintering over the hybrids, so I usually treat them as annuals. A rose must have fragrance to get my nod. Roses make us feel better just by their sheer beauty and aroma. Rose petal oil is very beneficial for the skin.

Parts used: Petals, hips and bark. Used as tea, tincture, and oil

Medicinal Uses: Rose petals and bark can be used to make rosewater for skin care and to stanch minor bleeding from scratches. Rose hips are known, primarily for their vitamin C content and were used to treat scurvy years ago. They also contain rather large amounts of vitamin A and smaller amounts of vitamin B3, vitamin D and vitamin E. Vitamin A is the skin vitamin and helps to regenerate skin cells, heal wounds, and minimize scars. Hips are a good source of carotenoids, flavonoids, polyphenols, citric acid, bioflavonoid, and zinc. Rose hips are thought to be anti-cancer, anti-depressant, antispasmodic, nervine, sedative and aphrodisiac. Rose hip tea is a mild diuretic and laxative. Hips are an immune booster and may prevent infection from viruses and bacteria. Studies to verify these uses are few and far between.

98

Rose petals are mildly sedative, antiseptic, and anti-parasitic. They are a mild laxative and a good supportive tonic for the heart. Also good for lowering cholesterol. The antiseptic nature of rose petals makes them a good treatment for wounds, bruises, rashes, and incisions. Rose petal tea is rich in gallic acid and is known to have anticancer, antimicrobial, anti-inflammatory, and analgesic effects.

Rose Hip Tea: Chop 2 heaping teaspoonfuls of rose hips (with or without seeds). Add hips and 1 cup boiling water to a cup and steep for 15 minutes. Strain and sweeten with honey as the tea is extremely tart. Tea works best if taken at bedtime.

Rose petal oil: 1 ounce rose petals to 7 ounces quality oil. Spread the petals out on a tray and let wilt overnight. Place in a blender with 2 tablespoons vodka. Blend until well macerated. Let sit overnight. Add the oil and blend on high for 3-5 minutes, until the oil is warm. Blend about 5 times over the next 48 hours. Strain through a muslin cloth into a sterile jar and store in a dark place.

Rosemary

(Rosmarinus officinalis)

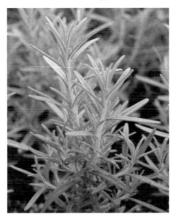

Rosemary is a member of the mint family along with oregano, thyme, basil, and lavender, hailing from the Mediterranean area. Can be sown indoors in sunny location or under plant grow lights eight weeks before last frost. Rosemary propagates well via stem cuttings too. Rosemary plants should be spaced between 18 and 24 inches (45 - 60 cm) apart in a light, well-drained soil or in containers. Prefers full sun and warmth. Allow soil to go dry between watering, then soak thoroughly.

Parts used: Leaves. Used as tea, liniment, tincture, and salve

Medicinal uses: Traditionally used to help alleviate muscle pain. Soups and teas can ease sinus pain. Stimulates circulation and acts as a tonic for the central nervous system. Much like peppermint, its scent improves memory and concentration as well as a being a mood booster. Some studies suggest that rosemary may significantly help prevent brain aging. Studies have shown that the carnosic and rosmarinic acids in rosemary have powerful antibacterial, antiviral, and antifungal properties. Consuming rosemary regularly can potentially help lower the risk of infection and help the immune system fight any infections that do occur. Also highly anti-oxidant. A report published in the *Journal of Food Science* revealed that adding rosemary extract to ground beef reduces the formation of cancer-causing agents that can develop during cooking.

Rosemary tea: bring 10 ounces of water to a boil. Place 1 teaspoon of rosemary leaves in a tea ball, in a cup and pour the water over. Let steep for 5-10 minutes, depending on how flavorful you prefer your tea.

Caution: Very high doses of rosemary leaves can cause vomiting, coma, spasms, and pulmonary edema, because of the volatile oils. Although this is rare.

Sage

(Salvia officinalis)

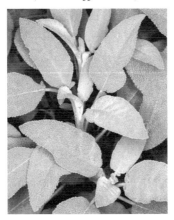

Sage is perennial in more temperate climates but is treated as an annual here in the interior. Sage can be grown from seeds, but the best way to grow high-quality sage is from cuttings from an established plant. Start the seeds/cuttings indoors 6 to 10 weeks before the last spring frost. Plant the seeds/cuttings in well-drained, sandy, loamy, soil 1 to 2 weeks before the last spring frost. Plant the seeds/cuttings 24 to 30 inches apart. For best growth, the soil should be between 60° and 70°F. Prefers a pH between 6.0 and 7.0. Resist the temptation to over-fertilize; the sage might grow a little faster, but its flavor will be less intense. Plant sage in medium to full sun. If you are growing sage indoors, place your pot near a sunny window. In the garden, plant near rosemary, cabbage, and carrots, but keep sage away from cucumbers.

Parts used: Leaves. Used as tea, decoction, tincture, salve

Medicinal Uses: Sage is a do-all, end-all herb. It has been used for thousands of years for improving memory and preventing age-related memory loss. Sage promotes calmness and increases contentment according to some studies. Sage extracts are used to alleviate the pain and inflammation of a sore throat. Tea or diluted tincture are also good for a mouthwash or gargle for sore throat. Studies in animal research have suggested that sage may stabilize blood sugar in chemically induced diabetes in rats. Sage also warrants further study as it appears to prevent skin cancer and kill colon cancer cells. Valuable antibacterial, antifungal and antiviral. Internally will fight infection and diminish secretions of all kinds, including perspiration and saliva. Tea or tincture is used for drying up milk production during weaning. Stimulates memory.

Caution: Do not use medicinally during pregnancy. Do not take medicinally on an ongoing basis.

Sage Tincture: Gather several handfuls of sage. Wash only if necessary, dry thoroughly. Chop the sage and place in a sterile pint jar. Cover with vodka or other high proof alcohol. Seal and shake the jar every day or so for 2-4 weeks. Strain and squeeze to get every possible bit of constituent. Pour into colored glass bottle. Use as a gargle for sore throat or take 1 teaspoonful at the first sign of a cold. Dilute with a little water rather than taking it straight.

Scullcap

(Scutellaria lateriflora)

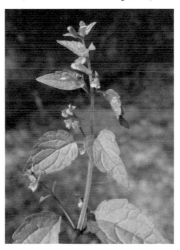

Scullcap is a hardy perennial, native to North America. It is a member of the mint family. It loves a wetland habitat and grows near marshes, meadows, and other wet habitats. The name refers to the flower's resemblance to helmets worn by European soldiers. To grow, refrigerate the seeds for a week before planting them in pots or flats. Press gently into the soil and mist with water. Cover container with plastic wrap and place in a warm sunny spot. Remove plastic as soon as leaves appear and mist lightly each day. Transfer seedlings to a shady spot in the garden. Keep moist. Harvest as they mature.

Parts used: Leaves, stems, and flowers. Used as tea and tincture.

Medicinal uses: A mild sedative that offers quick relief from anxiety, nerve pain, and nervous tension. Also helpful with uneasy feelings around menopause. Used for centuries by Native Americans to treat menstrual disorders, nervousness, digestive and kidney problems.

Skullcap can be used as a hot infusion by pouring 1 cup of boiling water over 1 -2 teaspoons of dried herb for 15 minutes or taken as a tincture extract. May help protect against neurological disorders such as Alzheimer's and Parkinson's. Recent research has revealed that skullcap contains the flavonoids baicalin, baicalein, wogonin and scutellarin as well as the amino acids glutamine, glutamate and GABA, which possibly attributes to its anxiolytic properties.

Caution: Do not take during pregnancy and or breastfeeding, or if you have liver disease, epilepsy, or a seizure disorder.

Spearmint

(Mentha spicata)

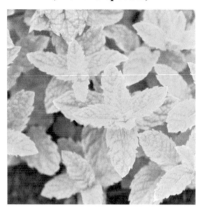

Spearmint is native to Europe and is closely related to peppermint. It grows well in the interior as an annual plant but be aware that most Menthas tend to be thugs and plan to take over the world. It is easily started from cuttings or runners. The adult plant in Fairbanks is usually about 18 inches tall and can spread 3-4 feet wide, unless pruned regularly. It is a pretty plant with spear shaped leaves and pinkish flower stalks.

Medicinal Uses: The leaves are the part of the plant used and contain many active ingredients similar to peppermint. The most active properties in spearmint are Mint L-carvone and limonene. Although spearmint has more limonene and less l-carvone than peppermint. That is why they taste different. It is used as a digestive aid and to control flatulence. It relieves nausea, cold symptoms, cramps headache, and indigestion. It is also applied topically, to the skin, to help reduce swelling due to nerve or muscle pain. Experiments with spearmint in the treatment of hirsutism (excessive hair growth) are ongoing as it shows some promise in alleviating this condition. Its other uses are similar to peppermint.

Spearmint Oil: Pack a jar with crushed spearmint leaves. Cover the leaves with olive oil. Place in the sun for 2 weeks or in a cool place for a month. Shake once a day. Strain the oil and store in a sterile jar or bottle in a dark, dry place. The oil will keep for up to 3 months, up to a year if refrigerated. Use topically.

St. John's Wort

(Hypericum perforatum)

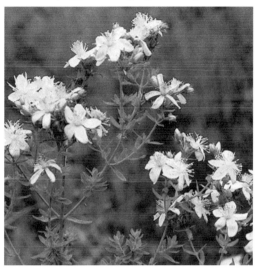

St. John's Wort was mainly used for magic potions during the Middle Ages. It grows well in sand, clay, rocky soil, or loam, and tolerates acidic to slightly alkaline pH. Adapts well to both moist and dry soil, and even tolerates occasional flooding. It also withstands drought but grows best with irrigation during prolonged dry spells. Growing St. John's wort herb in a location with too much sun can lead to leaf scorch, while too much shade reduces the number of flowers. The best conditions are bright morning sunlight and a little shade in the hottest part of the afternoon. If your soil isn't particularly fertile, prepare the bed before transplanting. Spread about 2 inches of compost or rotted manure over the area and dig it in to a depth of at least 8 inches. Transplant the plants into the garden, setting them at the height at which they grew in their containers. Space them 24 to 36 inches apart. Water slowly and deeply after planting and keep the soil moist until the transplants are well-established. Makes an attractive ground cover and soil stabilizer. Once established, the plants need no care, and this makes them ideal for out-of-the-way locations. You can also use as an edging, in containers, rock gardens and foundation plantings. Can self-seed.

Parts used: Flowers and upper leaves. Used as tea, tincture and infused oil.

Medicinal uses: Effective as an anti-depressant. Can help alleviate anxiety and symptoms associated with mild depression. Also a strong antiviral that can shorten the duration of cold sores when applied topically. Other topical uses include treatment of arthritis, fibromyalgia, muscle aches, and sciatica.

Caution: Do not take if taking MAOI or SSRI medications. Can weaken antidepressants, birth control pills, Cyclosporine (used to prevent organ rejection), Digoxin, Oxycodone, some HIV drugs, some cancer medications (including irinotecan), and Warfarin. Side effects are minor and uncommon, but they can include upset stomach, dry mouth, headache, fatigue, dizziness, confusion, or sexual dysfunction. When applying oil to fair skin, keep out of sun, as it may cause a sensitivity to sunlight. Wear gloves to harvest and do not touch eyes or mucous membranes. St. John's Wort is a stimulant and may worsen feelings of anxiety in some people.

Thyme

(Thymus vulgaris)

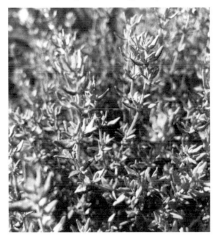

Thyme is a perennial in the more temperate zones but only occasionally for us. It is a low growing spreading mass of tiny leaves. There are about 350 varieties of thyme in existence, but only some are aromatic and flower. English thyme and lemon thyme are too very popular culinary thymes. Thyme is highly aromatic and attracts bees and other pollinators. They are easy to tuck in small spots and are said to repel pest and beetles on brassicas. It is easiest to purchase starts or propagate cuttings and transplant them. They germinate slowly and unevenly. Begin harvesting the tops when 4-6 inches tall and keep harvesting regularly to keep them from becoming to woody.

Parts used: Leaves. Used as tea, tincture, poultice

Medicinal Uses: Thymol is the major essential oil in thyme. It is antibacterial as well as anti-fungal and is effective in the treatment of bronchitis, whooping cough, and upper respiratory diseases. It is also known for battling cancer. Thyme has one of the highest levels of phenolic antioxidants among herbs. It contains vitamins A, K, C. folic acid and B complex plus potassium, iron, calcium, manganese, magnesium, and selenium. A small amount steeped as tea is effective. I use a basil, thyme, honey tea for coughs associated with colds and flu. It works at least as well as some of the OTC cough syrups do.

Caution: Generally considered safe but regular overuse may result in abnormal menstrual cycles.

Tea: Place 1 tsp. basil and thyme in a tea ball and pour boiling water over the herbs. Steep for 10-15 minutes. Add honey to taste. Sip to control coughing.

Thyme Cough Syrup: 1/3 cup thyme or lemon thyme, 1/3 cup marshmallow root, 1/3 cup slippery elm bark, 2 cups (or more) raw honey. Mix herbs and add to a jar big enough to hold the herbs and honey. Cover the herbs with honey, making sure they are completely saturated. Cover with a tight lid and shake. Place in a cool dark place and each morning turn the jar upside down. Each evening, turn it right side up. Do this for 30 days, then strain the herbs. This is made easier by warming the honey slightly in a bowl of hot water. Once the herbs have been strained, and the honey is in a clean container, store in the refrigerator for up to a year.

Tulsi or Holy Basil

(Ocimum sanctum syn. O.tenuiflorum)

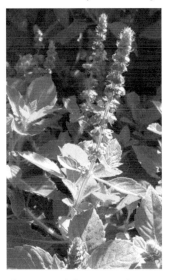

Holy Basil has been used for centuries as a medicinal in India and Asia. Studies on Holy Basil (O.tenuiflorum) have shown that its many phytonutrients and antioxidants may prevent or treat many illnesses. It is considered a super-food and is included in kitchen gardens, in pots beside doorways or any place to have it readily available. To get an early start, plant seeds indoors in flats, several weeks before the final frost. Transplant the seedlings to a garden bed when they are about 3 inches tall. Loves full sun at least six hours each day; more sun is preferable. Work in organic compost to a depth of 12 inches. Plant directly in the garden at any point after the final spring frost. Press seeds into place 1/4 inch deep in the soil so that they do not float away when watered. Cover the seeds with soil, and water the soil. As the plants develop, thin to 18 inches. Water plants enough to keep them moist but avoid excess irrigation. All basil varieties are subject to "damping-off" disease triggered by too much moisture. When the seedlings are 3 inches tall, spread coarse mason sand to a depth of 2 inches over the soil around the plants. Sand mulch reduces weeds, controls moisture and moderate temperature fluctuations. Clip off the central stem of each plant about six weeks after the seedlings

112

sprout. Leave only two leaf sets on each stem to encourage the development of leafy lateral branches. Harvest some holy basil leaves when the leaves become plentiful. Remove some leaves several times each week to encourage other leaves to grow. Leaves are most pungent just as a plant starts to bud. Pinch off buds before they flower to keep the plant productive. When plant's flowers bloom, the plant stops producing leaves. Holy basil also grows well in containers on a deck or in pots in a sunny window.

Parts used: Leaf and flowering tops, dried seeds, and dried roots. Used as tea, decoction, and tinctures.

Medical uses: An adaptogen that helps reduce physical and psychological effects of stress, enhances physical and mental endurance by optimizing assimilation of oxygen and nutrients to bloodstream. Strong antioxidant that helps prevent cancer, heart disease, arthritis, diabetes, and dementia. Helps normalize blood sugar, blood pressure, and reduces LDL cholesterol. Also helps with cough, colds, flu and fever. Tulsi has been found to protect organs and tissues against chemical stress from industrial pollutants and heavy metals. Its strong broad-spectrum antimicrobial activity, which includes activity against a range of human and animal pathogens, suggest it can be used as a hand sanitizer, mouthwash, and water purifier as well as a wound healer.

Valerian

(Valeriana officinalis)

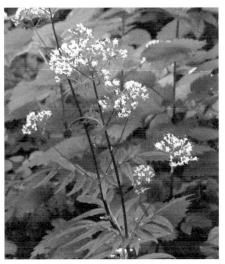

Valerian is perennial in the Fairbanks area. If you know someone who has some, they will most likely share their new seedlings that pop up everywhere. If you are planting seeds, sow them into warm soil after all danger of frost has passed. Keep seedlings watered. Can grow to heights of 5 feet. It emits a pleasant vanilla/cinnamon-like fragrance. Harvest roots in fall.

Parts used: roots. Used as tea, powdered in capsules, and tincture.

Medicinal uses: Natural sleep aid and can be used with other remedies when pain is preventing sleep. Non-habit forming. Releases smooth muscles, so also useful for menstrual cramps.

Caution: Generally considered safe but can act as a stimulant in some people and may not be safe if you are pregnant or breastfeeding. Side effects such as headache, dizziness, stomach problems or sleeplessness are rare but have occurred.

Yarrow

(Achillea millefolium)

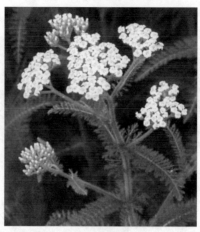

Grows wild and is easily grown in a garden. Sow seeds and water. A self-seeding perennial that gives a harvest year after year. Begin harvesting as soon as the plants mature, picking the leaves and flowers in the early morning and drying them right away.

Parts used: Leaves and flowers. Used as tea, tincture, salve and poultice.

Medicinal uses: A natural styptic, a substance that stops bleeding by contracting body tissue and healing injured blood vessels. Encourages clotting and helps disinfect minor wounds. Use as poultice. Tincture or tea can help reduce heavy menstrual bleeding.

Caution: Do not take internally during pregnancy or lactation. It is reported to be an abortifacient and to affect the menstrual cycle. Can cause a rash in some who are allergic to plants in the Asteraceae family.

Always do your own research to see what works for you. Here are some websites to investigate for cross referencing:

https://medlineplus.gov/druginfo/herb_All.html

https://nccih.nih.gov/health/herbsataglance.htm

https://www.mskcc.org/cancer-care/diagnosis-treatment/symptom-management/integrative-medicine/herbs/about-herbs

https://altnature.com/

More Recipes

Calendula Skin Salve

Melt 1/8 cup grated beeswax in the top of a double boiler. Remove from heat and add ½ cup calendula infused oil. Heat should never exceed 105 to 110 degrees. Stir in 20 drops of lavender essential oil. Pour into a clean jar or tin. Use to relieve rashes and chaffing.

Bruise Blend

10 drops helichrysum essential oil

3 drops lemongrass essential oil

8 drops lavender essential oil

3 drops geranium essential oil

3 drops cypress essential oil

36 drops fractionated coconut oil or other carrier oil

Drop into roller ball bottle and shake. Apply to bruise several times a day until you see a change.

Herbal Vinegar for Colds and Flu

3 tablespoons minced onion

3 tablespoons minced garlic

3 tablespoons grated fresh ginger

3 tablespoons grated horseradish

3 tablespoons mustard seed

3 tablespoons black peppercorns

1 or more whole chilies (1 tsp. dried)

1 cup apple cider vinegar

1/3 cup honey

Put onion, garlic, horseradish, mustard seeds, peppercorns, and chilies in a sterile glass jar. Stir until well mixed. Pour vinegar over mix to fill jar. Should be about 1 inch of vinegar above the mix. Cap with a plastic lid (metal will rust). Let sit 2-4 weeks, shaking daily. After 2-4 weeks, strain through cheesecloth or muslin into a sterile glass container. Squeeze the cloth to extract all of the liquid. Add honey to help preserve it and to help it taste a little better. Label and date before storing. Keeps up to 2 years.

Take ½ to 1 tsp every hour until cold or flu symptoms subside. Makes 2 cups

Note: Apple cider vinegar has both antibiotic and antiseptic properties that may neutralize toxins in the body.

Lotions & Potions

Introduction

We started this project with me kicking and screaming my total lack of interest in this. Marsha convinced me to at least give it a try, so here we are. When I began to see the impact of the chemicals that I and my family were exposed to on a daily basis, I saw the sense in going ahead with this. We hope that you will be able to reduce your exposure to some harmful chemicals in your cosmetics, drinks, and cleaning products.

We weren't born knowing this stuff. We spend hours researching, checking facts, trying recipes, and getting them down on paper. We've had some failures, some things that needed adjustments and some that neither of us liked, but through it all, we've learned a lot and had fun. This is our hope for you too. And that you will be able to enjoy a less chemically dependent life. Here are a few simple things for you to try.

COSMETICS

Where Do I Start?

Take a look at the products you are currently using. Are there things listed that you can't pronounce and have no idea what they are? That's a clue that they may not be a very healthy choice. You can check out those chemicals at ewg.org to see if they are on the list of hazardous substances. If they are, you can develop a plan to eliminate as many as possible from your home. Many of the chemicals found in cosmetics and cleaning products are hormone disrupters. These can have negative effects on adults and can be seriously injurious to children.

Some to watch for:

Poloxamer

Retinyl

Propylparaben

Octinoxate

Butylphenyl Methyl Propional

Oxybenzone

Many of these are known carcinogens, some have adverse effects on lungs, some are endocrine disrupters, and some cause severe allergic response. I found these in foundation makeup, lip balm with sunscreen and facial cleansers. I also looked at my shampoo bottle. I purposely used well known beauty shop brands to try to avoid some of the chemicals. It didn't work. My particular brand got a "C" rating for its chemical makeup. There are others on the market that would be safer, you just have to consciously look. You might make a list of the worst chemicals and take it to the store with you. Don't fall for the ALL-NATURAL banners, that is not a regulated claim. Read the ingredient list and if you can't pronounce them or it is on the nasty list, pass it up. Let's work on getting cleansing products and creams that will not have all these chemicals in them. Check out www.ewg.org.

If we can clean our faces with almond oil and hot water and get smoother, softer skin, then why buy expensive chemical products to get similar results. Many of the cosmetics that we have developed for our use are made with essential oils rather than fresh or dried herbs. Essential oils are a more concentrated form and are easier to measure for aroma and strength. It is possible to infuse oils with fresh or dried herbs prior to beginning a cream too.

Here are some herbs to consider for DIY cosmetics and their effects:

Relaxing herbs: Chamomile, hops, jasmine, citrus flowers, valerian and lavender

Stimulating herbs: Basil, bay, eucalyptus, fennel, lemon balm, lemon verbena, rosemary

Soothing herbs: Apple mint, chervil, lavender, lemon balm, rose, mint, thyme

Mature skin herbs: Lemon verbena, rose, geranium

Dry skin herbs: Borage, parsley, sorrel

Oily skin herbs: Calendula, sage, yarrow

We have included some of our tried and successful experiments for you to try. There are also thousands of recipes available on the internet for you to pick and choose for yourself.

RECIPES

Rosewater

Rose water is a refreshing spray and may calm skin irritations.

1-2 cups fresh rose petals

1 cup water

Wash rose petals. Inspect for bugs or dirt, then wash again if necessary. Put the rose petals in a saucepan and cover with the water Heat on low only to simmering and simmer 15-20 minutes. Cool completely and strain through cheesecloth, squeezing rose petals to extract as much constituent as possible. Put in clean, sterile spray bottle. Spray on skin.

Rosewater Toner

3/4 cup fresh rose petals (2 Tablespoons dried)

1 cup white vinegar (herbal vinegar works)

1 cup rose water

Mix rose petals and vinegar in glass jar. Let sit for 2 weeks or more. The longer it sits the stronger it gets, up to about 4 weeks. Strain through cheesecloth, squeezing to extract the juice. Add rose water and mix well. Spray or pat onto skin with cotton pad.

Rosewater Emollient

2 tablespoons rosewater

1 tablespoon witch hazel

2 tablespoons glycerin

1 ½-2 tablespoon almond oil, jojoba oil, or nurturing oil of choice

Mix all ingredient together in a tightly capped bottle. Will separate between uses, so shake before use.

Body Butter For Dry Skin

¼ cup grated cocoa butter

1 tablespoon beeswax pearls or grated

1 tablespoon coconut oil

2 tablespoons sesame oil

1 tablespoon avocado oil or almond oil

Melt cocoa butter and beeswax in a double boiler or in the microwave, just until both are melted. Add the rest of the oils, stirring to combine well. Pour into a container and let cool completely. Makes 4 oz.

ETC Body Cream

1 cup aloe vera gel

1/3 cup coconut oil

1 tsp vitamin E oil

¾ cup almond oil

1 tablespoon lanolin (op.)

1 to 1 ½ tablespoons (1/2 to ¾ oz.) beeswax pearls or grated

Up to 1 ½ teaspoons essential oil of choice

(Lavender and geranium are good for your skin)

Place aloe gel, lanolin, and vitamin E oil in a blender or food processor, or use an immersion blender. Put coconut oil and beeswax in a 2 cup Pyrex measuring cup, microwave or heat double boiler style, stirring occasionally until the beeswax is fully melted. Stir in the almond oil. Turn blender on slow speed and pour in oils in a slow thin stream. When it is the consistency of mayonnaise, add essential oils and pulse to mix. Transfer to a jar quickly before the cream starts to set up.

Geranium Facial Wipes

We keep these in the refrigerator in the summer to cool off and refresh.

8 drops Geranium Essential Oil

1 ounce witch hazel

12 heavy duty paper towels or paper hand towels

Mix essential oil and witch hazel together. Put paper towels in a resealable bag and pour the witch hazel mix over the towels. Make sure the towels are saturated. Refrigerate until needed. Take one towel and wipe your face to cool off. You can use any essential oil but geranium and lavender are cooling.

Teeth Cleaning Powder

3 tablespoons bentonite clay

3 teaspoons baking soda

1 teaspoon fine grain salt

Peppermint oil or extract to taste

Combine all ingredients and mix thoroughly. Store in a jar and use in place of toothpaste.

Natural Tooth Paste

2 tablespoons coconut oil

2 teaspoons salt

2 tablespoons baking soda

Peppermint extract to taste

Mix all ingredients together and store in an airtight container.

Natural Deodorant

Try this non-aluminum and inexpensive version:

2 ½ tablespoons coconut oil, warmed to a liquid state

2 tablespoons baking soda

2 ½ tablespoons cornstarch or arrowroot powder

5-8 drops of your favorite essential oil

(rosemary or basil are nice antibacterials with a pleasant scent)

Mix all ingredients together and let solidify. Stirring occasionally so they don't separate. Store in a jar. To use, just dab under arms and rub in.

Another natural deodorant:

This one can be put into a twist-tube or a jar. It is firmer than the above recipe but will soften in warm weather.

1/3 cup coconut oil

1 1/2 teaspoons grated bees wax or pearls (more if you want it firmer)

1-2 tablespoons baking soda (depending on if you are sensitive to soda)

3 tablespoons cornstarch or arrowroot powder

1 1/2 teaspoons bentonite clay

5-8 drops rosemary, sandalwood, or lavender essential oil or your favorite.

Melt bees wax and add the coconut oil, melting it too. Add remaining ingredients, except the essential oils. Let cool, stirring occasionally until it becomes a pudding-like consistency. Add the essential oil and spoon into deodorant containers or jar. Let harden.

Foot Cream

1 oz. grated beeswax or pearls

2 oz. cocoa butter

2 oz. shea butter

2 oz. coconut oil

2 oz. sesame oil

1 oz. vegetable glycerine

About 1/3 cup water

5-10 drops essential oils

(tea tree, lavender, eucalyptus, thyme, or rosemary – all one oil or a comination)

Melt beeswax, cocoa butter, and shea butter. Blending with an immersion blender or hand mixer, slowly add coconut oil, sesame oil, and glycerine. Add water in a thin stream until smooth and creamy. Blend in essential oils. Put into jars and let set.

Silky Body Butter

6 tablespoons or 3 oz. green tea or chamomile tea

1/4 teaspoon citric acid dissolved in tea (a skin softener, op.)

1 tablespoon chopped beeswax or beeswax pearls

1 tablespoon cocoa butter, grated

1 tablespoon Shea butter

6 tablespoons coconut oil

1 1/2 teaspoons liquid lanolin

6 tablespoons or 3 liquid oz. grapeseed, olive or a combination of nourishing oils. (almond, avocado, jojoba)

2 tablespoons vegetable glycerin

1 teaspoon vitamin E

10-20 drops essential oil of choice

Make tea and measure out 6 tablespoons. Add citric acid, if desired and stir to dissolve. Set aside. Melt beeswax over low heat. Add cocoa butter, shea butter and coconut oil. Melt all together. Remove from heat and add liquid lanolin and nourishing oils. Blend with a hand blender or with a mixer. Add in vegetable glycerin, vitamin E and blend again. With blender or mixer on, gradually add tepid tea. (If it has gotten cold, warm it slightly or it will coagulate the beeswax.) Blend until all is combined and is silky smooth. Add essential oils if you would like a scented body butter.

Chocolate Lip Balm

1 ½ teaspoons grated cocoa butter

½ teaspoon grated dark chocolate

½ teaspoon coconut oil

1-2 drops essential oil* (op.)

Combine ingredients in a microwave bowl or double boiler. Heat gently until melted and liquid is smooth. Pour into small jar or lip balm tube. Allow to cool completely. *Essential oils to try: orange, mint, or lavender.

Balancing Bath Salts (single use)

3 tablespoons sea salt

1 tablespoon citric acid powder

2 tablespoons baking soda

8 drops essential oil

Small jar

Choose one or more oils from these: bergamot, frankincense, geranium, lavender palmarosa, rose, or rosewood.

Combine sea salt, baking soda, citric acid powder and oils in a jar. Seal and shake to mix thoroughly. Add to running hot water in a bathtub.

Relaxing Bath Salts

3 cups Epsom salts

3 cups table or sea salt

2 cups baking soda

Lavender essential oil or oil of your choice

Mix salt and baking soda in a large bowl. Put 1/2 cup salt mix in smaller bowl, add lavender essential oil until you reach desired fragrance. Stir until well mixed. You could add lavender food coloring at this point, if desired. Make sure color is distributed throughout the mix. Add lavender salt mix to large bowl of salts and stir until fragrance and color are equally distributed throughout the salts. Be sure to stir up the bottom of the bowl as oil and color tend to cling there. Pour into jars and seal with airtight lids. Use ¼ cup salts under running warm or hot bath water.

Drinks

Our Liquid Life

Drinks are as common as your morning tea or coffee and as rare as those cute little umbrella drinks we sip on vacation. We all have our specialties that make life happier. For some of us our morning tea or coffee is the jumpstart to the day and for some of us an alcohol beverage at the end of the day is the frosting to a good day.

We read that soda is a leading cause of obesity in the United States both because of the sugar content, and the chemical compounds, plus the quantity that we consume. We worry that our kids and grandkids are going to have serious health problems as a result of some of these factors.

Some things we cannot fix. Drinks, however, are in the fix-it category. You can make homemade soda that is yummy with less sugar and no chemicals. You can carbonate juices to increase the nutritive value of what you drink while making them fun. Herbs for flavoring will also increase the nutritional value. Kombucha and kefir are somewhat healthy alternatives, but the store brands have quite a bit of sugar and they are very expensive. You can make these at home too.

Let's look at some things we might do to improve our drinking life.

Recipes

Teas

You can use almost any herb to make tea. You may make it plain with only 1 herb or add herbs to black or green tea, steeping this combination 3-5 minutes. You can also blend herbs to create your own special signature tea. Experiment to find what you like. Start your experience using 1-2 teaspoons of dried herb or 1-2 tablespoons fresh herb in a tea ball, bag, or sieve. Crush the herbs to release the oils and add to 1 cup of boiling water. Steep for 5-15 minutes. Herbs may become bitter if steeped too long. You may also have to adjust the amount of herb to suit your taste. Compost spent herbs or tea leaves.

Citrus herbs blend with almost anything and do well as additions to black or green tea. You might find lemon herbs, green tea, and ginger to be tasty and refreshing. they also have many healthy constituents.

Some herbs to try for tea are: anise hyssop, lavender, lemon balm, scented mints, marjoram, lemon thyme, lemon verbena , scented geraniums, mints, sage, lemon grass, ginger, chamomile, and scented basils. You can also mix and match. Our favorites vary with seasons and whims.

Shrubs

Shrubs or drinking vinegars had their origin in colonial America. They are a mix of vinegar, fruit, herbs, and sweeteners that results in a tart, tangy syrup concentration. They are an easy, fun project using your fruits and herbs to make specialty drinks. There are now shrub bars around the country with varieties lining shelves as the combinations are endless.

Aromatics, such as herbs, impart essential flavor that enhances the fruit base. Basil and sage stand on their own against the strong flavors of the fruits. The fruit can overwhelm the milder herb flavors so try combinations of herbs to create signature flavors.

Always use fresh healthy herbs and don't throw them away when you drain them from the shrub. Use them in marinades or vinaigrettes.

There are a gazillion recipes out there . Some with kale, tomato, rhubarb or jalapeno, but I think we'll stick with herb/fruit shrubs. You don't have to use perfect fruit for a shrub, after all you are going to macerate so blemishes won't show. Just don't use spoiled or moldy fruits. Use nice ripe, juicy ones. Citrus fruits generally don't lend themselves to shrubs because combined with the vinegar, the final syrup may be a bit to mouth puckering.

Mash, grate, or mince the fruits so the most flavor and juice will be extracted.

Shrubs have a long shelf life due to the vinegar's acetic acid. The vinegar you choose is a matter of personal taste.

White vinegar does not impart other flavors, but it does have a much bigger bite than some like champagne, un-seasoned rice vinegar, white wine, or red wine vinegars. Apple cider vinegar also has it's own flavor that may enhance or overpower fruit and/or herbs depending on which ones you choose. Balsamic vinegar goes well with cherries or berries, but it has a pretty strong flavor, so you may want to combine it with another vinegar. Red wine vinegar intensifies the color of red fruits, like strawberries, cherries or raspberries.

Your choice of sweetener is entirely up to you, The most common shrubs use granulated or raw cane sugar. Demara, turbinado, and muscovado will change the flavor a bit but will work just fine. Honey, maple or agave syrups will each add a distinctive taste to your shrub but will dilute the taste of the fruit with their volume.

Here is a basic recipe to play with:

133

2 parts mashed fresh or frozen fruit

1 part sugar

1 part vinegar

You can also add:

¼ cup flower petals, like roses, lavender, nasturtiums or elderberry blossoms.

¼ cup fresh herbs, such as basil, thyme, rosemary, mint, dill, tarragon, or fennel

1 tablespoon freshly grated turmeric, ginger, or chopped lemongrass

There are 2 methods of making shrubs – cold and hot.

Cold Process Method: Wash and sterilize a mason jar and lid in a canner or large pot. Macerate the herbs and fruit with a mortar or the back of a spoon in a bowl. Measure sweetener and add to the fruit and herbs, Spoon mixture into the hot mason jar. Refrigerate. Fruit/herb mixtures should wait 48 hours before adding the vinegar.

Thoroughly combine the vinegar and fruit mix, seal and return to the refrigerator. They should rest in the fridge for 2 to 4 weeks before decanting. In "herbs only" shrubs add the vinegar immediately. Herb only shrubs should sit undisturbed for up to a month. At the end of the resting period, strain the shrub through cheesecloth to remove the fruits and herbs. Return the shrub to a clean, sterile mason jar and refrigerate. Be sure to label, label, label.

Basil will turn black and slimy in the cold process. You can make an infused vinegar with basil and add to your fruit though. We prefer using the hot process method for anything with basil.

Hot Process Method: Sterilize jars and lids. Place sweetener in a saucepan and cover with an equal amount of water (1:1). Heat on medium until sweetener is dissolved, stirring constantly. Reduce heat to medium low and add prepared fruit and herbs. Simmer for 20 to 25 minutes. Remove from heat and allow to cool. Strain fruit and herbs through cheesecloth. Add vinegar to reserved liquid and put in sterilized jar. Label and refrigerate.

Shrubs keep in the refrigerator for 3-6 months.

Preparing drinks with a shrub:

Drizzle a couple tablespoons (or to taste) of shrub syrup into a glass of juice, water, soda water, or spirits (vodka). It can also be added to sparkling wine, iced tea and even beer.

You can make a quick salad dressing by whisking 2 tablespoons shrub to 4-6 tablespoons extra virgin olive oil. Add salt, pepper, and fresh minced garlic to taste.

You can use it as a drizzle over ice cream or cheesecake.

Some good combinations for shrubs are:

1 cup fresh lemon verbena, 1 cup fresh thyme leaves, 1 cup sweetener and 1 cup white wine vinegar.

2 cups fresh sage leaves, 1/2 to 1 cup honey, 1 cup apple cider vinegar

1 cup fresh strawberries, 1/2 cup fresh basil leaves, 1/2 to 1 cup sugar, 1 cup vinegar

1 cup fresh blueberries, 1/2 cup anise hyssop leaves, peel of 1 lemon, 1/2 to 1 cup sugar, 1 cup vinegar

These all make approximately 1 pint finished shrub syrup.

Other Drinks

You can make homemade sodas with fruit flavored syrups and lemon juice added to seltzer water, sparkling water, or club soda. Fill with ice and top off with an herb garnish or a little umbrella.

Water kefir and kombucha are both high on the health list right now. You can make both at home with a little effort. Both require "starters" that you can purchase at the health food store or get from a friend who is already making them.

Water Kefir

Two or more teaspoons hydrated water kefir grains, 1/4 cup sugar (unprocessed is nice) per quart of non-chlorinated, filtered, water. Do not use honey, as it will affect the beneficial bacteria in the kefir grains!

Dissolve the sugar in a small amount of hot water in a jar. When sugar is dissolved, add cool water to fill the jar. Mixture should be at room temperature. Add the hydrated water kefir grains. Cover with a towel, coffee filter or cheesecloth and put a rubber band around to keep out bugs or children. Keep at 70 to 75 degrees for 24 to 48 hours. The longer it sits the more the sugar ferments out. Don't leave longer than 48 hours. After your chosen time, strain the water kefir, grains through a bamboo or mesh strainer (don't use metal if you can avoid it) into a clean sterile jar You can go back to the beginning and start a new process with the hydrated water kefir grains. To carbonate the water kefir, pour a couple of ounces of grape, pomegranate, apple, or cherry juice into the strained kefir. Citrus juice does not work well. Once the juice is added, cover the jar/s tightly with an airtight lid and leave on the counter an additional 1 to 3 days before drinking or refrigerating.

Water kefir can be flavored after it has become fizzy with dried or fresh fruit, herbs, flavoring extracts, or fruit juices. Dried fruit can soak for up to a week, but fresh fruit must be changed every day.

Kombucha

Bring 1 gallon of distilled or filtered water to a boil in a clean container. The purity of the water will determine the lifespan of your culture. Add 1 cup organic sugar and simmer for 10 minutes or until sugar is completely dissolved. Turn off the heat and add 8 tea bags or 6 teaspoons black or green tea in a tea ball. Cool to room temperature.

Once the sugar/tea mixture has cooled you need to inoculate it with the kombucha cultures. The culture is called a SCOBY. You will save your SCOBY from each new batch along with about 2 cups of the old tea as a starter. This ensures that the ph is low and the cultures will be able to compete with any foreign cultures or molds that may be present. Put the white, creamy side of the SCOBY facing up in the jar.

If you forgot to save starter tea or just got a SCOBY from a friend, you can use 1 cup of organic vinegar as a starter for the first batch. Add both the starter tea (vinegar) and SCOBY to the sweetened tea solution.

Now the inoculated tea solution must sit in a warm, dark place, undisturbed for five to ten days so the fermentation process is completed. The tea prefers a temperature between 70 and 85 degrees to ferment. Temperature will determine the length of time it takes for your tea to be ready. After five days start checking to see if the tea is ready. The easiest way to tell is by taste and smell. Pull a small sample from the side of the jar with a straw. Try not to disturb the new SCOBY growing on top of the solution. It should have a slight vinegary smell and be slightly carbonated. If it still smells sweet and/or is flat, then give it a few more days. The taste should be fizzy, semi-sweet, and similar to apple cider in taste. The longer the tea sits the more pronounced the sharp vinegar taste will be, but this would contain a higher amount of beneficial medicinal properties. Gently remove the SCOBY and strain into sterile jars or bottles. At this point you can add fruit or fruit juice and let sit at room temp a day or two. You can choose to strain the fruit or not, but refrigerate to keep it from turning into vinegar.

Here are some notes from dietitian Maxine Smith, RD, LD, of the Cleveland Clinic:

"Some of kombucha's health benefits are similar to those of other fermented foods, like yogurt, kefir and raw (live) fermented pickles or sauerkraut," Smith says. "But it also has others — specific bioactive compounds — that are unique to kombucha."

Much of kombucha's gut-friendly accolades are likely due to the tea itself, and the polyphenols it contains.

"Polyphenols are known to act as strong antioxidants in the body and decrease inflammation, which is the root cause of many diseases and conditions," she explains. "And the fermentation process actually increases the amount of polyphenols." Kombucha also provides B vitamins, a handful of essential minerals, organic acids (Think: like when vinegar ferments) such as acetic, glucuronic and D-Saccharic acids. These acids, Smith says, have been shown to be antimicrobial, so they fight against bacterial growth. They can also promote detoxification by helping the liver get rid of undesired compounds that it has to process. Last, these acids help transport polyphenols in the body. Since some of those acids are produced from ethanol, Smith adds, it's worth noting that kombucha contains low levels of alcohol, usually ranging from 0.5 percent upwards to 3 percent. (To put that in perspective, your average craft beer clocks in at just under 6 percent.)

But just how beneficial is kombucha? "There aren't a lot of good quality, robust studies to support a lot of kombucha's hype, but the compounds it contains have been associated in some studies* with lowering cholesterol, lowering blood sugar, antimicrobial action, decreased rates of cancer, and improvement of liver and GI function.

Not suggested for pregnant females or children. So should those with certain chronic diseases (particularly liver or kidney disease or HIV), compromised immune systems and alcohol dependency. Suggested amount to drink is 4-12 ounces. Drinking too much kombucha could potentially lead to reactions like headache, nausea, GI distress or going into ketoacidosis (a medical emergency where there's too much acid in your blood), Smith continues.

*https://www.tandfonline.com/doi/full/10.1080/19476337.2
017.1410499

Herbal Booze

Basic Recipe: 3 parts alcohol of choice (vodka, rum, brandy, or gin) to 1 part fruit and small handful of herbs. Use glass or ceramic containers. Place fruit and herbs in the jar, pour in alcohol. Soak for 12 to 48 hours. Strain through a coffee filter or several layers of cheesecloth. Press the fruit lightly to extract as much liquid alcohol and fruit juice as possible. Store in refrigerator.

Herbed Vodka: Put a small handful of fresh herb (dill, parsley, oregano, and or/thyme) in a glass container. Cover with vodka. Allow to steep for 12-48 hours. Strain and refrigerate or freeze. May add a jalapeno pepper for some spice. Use for Bloody Marys.

Minty Rum: Put a small handful of fresh mint in a jar, cover with rum. Soak for 12 to 48 hours. Strain. Use for mojitos or minty rum & coke.

Vanilla Whiskey: Soak 1 or 2 vanilla beans in 2 cups of quality whiskey for 1 to 2 weeks, Remove vanilla beans and use for Irish coffee.

Cucumber Vodka: Soak cucumber slices, skin and all in vodka 24 hours, Do not soak longer as the cucumber will get bitter. You may add hot peppers, dill, or tarragon to the mix. Strain and store in the refrigerator. Cucumber will add lots of water so drink quickly as it is not shelf stable. Drink over ice on hot days.

Herbal Party Bar

Entertaining can be a bit of a hassle when you need to set up drinks for a large group. It doesn't have to be that way. You can prep the following ingredients, arrange them in a delicious array and let your guest help themselves. Make a couple of syrups first.

Citrus Spice Syrup: Bring 2 cups water, 2 cups sugar, peel from 2 oranges, and 1 lemon, 6 whole cloves and 2 cinnamon sticks to boil over medium high heat until sugar dissolves. Reduce heat and simmer 10 minutes. Cover and steep for 1 hour. Strain into a clean jar or small pitcher and refrigerate. Keeps up to 1 week.

Ginger Syrup: Bring 2 cups water, 2 cups Sugar and a 6-inch piece of ginger to a boil. Reduce to simmer and cook about 2 hours. Let cool, strain, and refrigerate up to 1 week. To increase the intensity of the ginger, you can leave the ginger in the syrup until ready to use.

Lemon Verbena Syrup: Bring 2 cups water, 1 2/3 cups sugar, and 20-30 lemon verbena leaves to a boil. Cover the pan, remove from heat and let steep 15 minutes. Strain and store in refrigerator for up to 4 days.

Place bowls of diced pineapple, mango, kiwi, peach, pear, banana, lime, lemon, orange, grapefruit, raspberries, blueberries, strawberries, mint, basil, lemon thyme, anise hyssop, and mints on a table. Arrange spiced syrups, sparkling water, club soda, ginger ale, crushed ice, measuring spoons and muddlers. (You may also provide gin, vodka, white wine, rum or tequila)

To use: place 2 tablespoons of fruit* and herb in a glass. Muddle with a spoon and add 2 tablespoons of syrup or to taste. Fill glass with crushed ice and top with water, sparkling water, or club soda. Booze should be added before the water or soda.

*Pineapple, lemon, mint, citrus syrup (Vodka)

*Mango, lime ginger syrup (gin)

*Watermelon, orange, (rum)

*Pineapple, mango, lemon thyme (white wine)

Add some finger foods and the party is ready.

Cleaning Green

Why Clean Green?

Marsha is much further along with cleaning without chemicals than I am. But I am learning to limit my use of products that contain words I cannot pronounce or have been highly processed. We really have very little knowledge of what many of these chemicals do, how they are absorbed by the body or what is absorbed. I do know that I have gotten rashes from using some cleaning products, over the course of the years. We are now hearing about endocrine disruption, cancers caused by or influenced by bisphenol-A (BPA), reproductive toxins and allergens. Not to mention what these chemicals do when they are released into our environment. We've listed some websites that are issuing warnings at the end of this section for you to see where we got some of our information.

The Environmental Protection Agency ranks indoor air pollution among the top environmental dangers and much of this pollution comes from common cleaning products and air fresheners. Immediate effects of exposure to these pollutants can include headaches, dizziness, fatigue, and irritation of the eyes, nose, and throat, as well as exacerbated symptoms of asthma and other respiratory illnesses. Long-term effects (following long or repeated exposure to indoor pollutants) include respiratory diseases, heart disease, and even cancer. The indoor pollutants that can cause these reactions are so common that the EPA strongly recommends everyone improve the air quality of their home, regardless of whether symptoms are currently present.

Words of caution. Despite the consequences of exposure to indoor air pollutants, the government doesn't regulate or assess the safety (or even the labeling) of the vast majority of cleaning products on the market. The EPA, meanwhile, only regulates cleaners that contain registered pesticides. This means that consumers are basically on their own when it comes to choosing safe cleaning products—a task that's *way* easier said than done.

141

We decided to try to come up with research and then develop recipes that would be as effective as the commercial chemical cleansers. Since we started this project, organics have become more available across the board. There are now some commercial products on the market that do a good job without the chemicals. Just be sure to read the labels as some replaced known chemical disrupters with some lesser-known ones.

We use vinegar, baking soda, washing soda and Castile soap mixes, with many variations. We continue to experiment with products, both ours and commercial, that have less impact on our bodies and the environment.

When you use a mix with washing soda, remember to wear rubber gloves. It is much stronger than baking soda and can cause irritation on your skin. Well, off to a cleaner, greener world. Before we get to the cleaning, let's check out some of the most common (and most useful) non-toxic and less toxic cleaning products.

Water

The most basic component of almost any cleaner is water. It dilutes the harsher cleaning agents. Some recipes call for distilled water to increase the longevity of the cleaner.

Baking Soda

Baking soda is a pantry staple with proven virus-killing abilities that also effectively cleans, brightens, and cuts through grease and grime.

It is a mild alkali, which helps grease and dirt dissolve in water. When not completely dissolved, baking soda acts as a gentle abrasive that can remove more stubborn dirt. On top of that, it's also an effective deodorizer.

142

Castile Soap

Castile soap is a style of soap that's made from 100 percent plant oils (meaning it uses no animal products or chemical detergents). Popularized by the Dr. Bronner's line of products, castile cuts through grease and cleans.

Vinegar

Thanks to its acidity, vinegar is nothing short of a cleaning wonder—it effectively (and gently!) eliminates grease, soap scum, and grime.

However, this acidity can also pose a danger to your floor. If you have natural stone flooring, you should not use a vinegar-based cleaner, as it can cause discoloration.

Lemon Juice

Natural lemon juice annihilates mold and mildew, cuts through grease, and shines hard surfaces (It also smells awesome.) Lemon juice is naturally acidic, making it tough on grease and hard water stains. Plus, that lemony scent is basically synonymous with "fresh." It's great for porcelain and ceramic tile, but make sure not to use it on flooring that can be damaged by acidity.

Olive Oil

This good-for-you cooking oil also works as a cleaner and polisher.

Borax

This is another alkali cleaner that helps to cut grease and oil. Once a common household cleaning supply, Borax, faded from popularity with the advent of modern cleaning products. However, it's making a comeback. This versatile powder can be used to create cleaning sprays, pastes, and scrubs. Some research suggests Borax can act as a skin and eye irritant. Use it wisely and don't ingest it.

Ammonia

As a cleaning component, ammonia is one of the toughest ingredients out there. It can tackle grease and grime for a streak-free shine. Because it's so potent, you should always be careful when using it. Wear gloves and make sure the area is well ventilated. Most importantly, **never mix ammonia with chlorine bleach**, as this will produce dangerous chlorine gas.

Rubbing Alcohol

We all know that alcohol works as a disin

fectant, so it only makes sense to use it to sanitize our floors. Rubbing alcohol, a.k.a. isopropyl alcohol also speeds up the evaporation rate to reduce the possibility of water damage from standing liquid on your floors.

Dish Soap

For a mild cleaner that is pH neutral, dish soap is the perfect ingredient. Simply mix it with water to clean rubber, tile, and more. Make sure to choose a dish soap without bleach, oils or moisturizers, since these additives can have unintended effects on your floor.

Essential Oils

Essential oils have gained popularity thanks to aromatherapy, but these naturally occurring plant compounds also make great scent additions to homemade cleaning products (particularly if you're not into the smell of vinegar). Essential oils are generally considered safe, but these extracts *can* trigger allergies—so keep this in mind when choosing scents.

A note on mixing products: Most of these ingredients can be used in combination with each other; however, many sources advise against mixing castile soap with vinegar or lemon juice. Since castile soap is basic (i.e., high on the pH scale) and vinegar and lemons are acidic, the products basically cancel each other out when used in combination (though it's fine to wash with a base— like castile soap—and rinse with an acid—like vinegar!).

Difference between washing soda and baking soda

The difference between baking soda and washing soda is water and carbon dioxide. Baking soda's chemical makeup is NaHCO3 (1 sodium, 1 hydrogen, one carbon, and 3 oxygen molecules). Washing soda's chemical makeup is Na2CO3 (2 sodium, 1 carbon, and 3 oxygen molecules). When baking soda is heated up to high temperatures, it breaks down to become washing soda, water steam, and carbon dioxide.

So, the steam and carbon dioxide are released during the cooking process, leaving you with… washing soda!

1) Washing Soda – Sodium Carbonate (Na2CO3) Otherwise known as soda ash, it is mainly used for **WASHING**. The compound is strong basic at pH

It is used as:

- water softener

- pH balancer

- photo developing agent in darkrooms (yes, people used to use chemicals to develop pictures and not just "upload" them to computers.)

- chemical to make chlorine less acidic and balance pH in pools

- to degrease, remove oil and wine stains

- to descale hard water for laundry, coffee pots and pipes

- polish silver

- But it is, **CAUSTIC and NOT EDIBLE.** And it's strongly advised to use gloves when cleaning with it and not inhale the particles.

2) Baking Soda – Sodium BiCarbonate (NaHCO3). Mainly used for **BAKING** and is a mild 'basic' with pH of 8.

It is used as:

- an antacid.

- a leavening agent as it reacts with acidic ingredients such as buttermilk and yogurt.

- cleaning agent and a deodorizer.

- an ingredient in toothpaste.

- a fire extinguisher in an emergency

And it is **SAFE TO EAT.** In short,

Washing Soda —> NOT EDIBLE

Baking Soda —> EDIBLE

Recipes

Simple All-Purpose Cleaner

Mix together equal parts vinegar and water in a spray bottle. If your countertop is made from marble, granite, or stone, skip the vinegar (its acidity is not good for these surfaces) and use rubbing alcohol or vodka instead.

Natural All-Purpose Cleaner

2 cups water

1 tablespoon baking soda

½ cup white vinegar

20-30 drops essential oil of choice

Add all ingredients to a spray bottle. Close the lid and shake gently. Shake before each use. Spray directly on cleaning surface and wipe or scrub gently. Always use first in a concealed place to make sure no damage is done to the materials. For this amount, I usually add up to 10 drops of a few different essential oils (they vary in concentration by kind).

**Alternatives: leave out the baking soda and/or add 1 Tbsp lemon juice.

**Here are some great disinfectant essential oil combinations to try:

- peppermint and tea tree

- lemongrass and lavender

- lavender and rosemary

- geranium and lime

- grapefruit, lemon, and lavender

- tea tree and orange

Homemade All-Purpose Floor Cleaner

2 cups warm water

1/2 cup white vinegar

1/4 cup rubbing alcohol

1/8 tsp dish soap (without bleach, oils or moisturizers)

(optional) 5-10 drops of essential oil or lemon juice

Combine all ingredients and spray or sponge on floors. Wipe dry.

Grapefruit Scouring Scrub Recipe

3 tablespoons dried, powdered grapefruit peels

3 tablespoons borax

5 tablespoons baking soda

Combine everything in a shaker (like an empty parmesan container) and shake well to combine it all. Use liberally wherever scouring is required. Be sure to rinse the scrub off well with a clean, wet sponge.

https://crunchybetty.com/the-great-grapefruit-scouring-scrub/

Citrus vinegar cleaner for grease and grime

Place citrus peels (any type) in a glass jar (pack fairly tightly) and cover with white vinegar. Place plastic lid on (or cover with plastic wrap) and let steep for two weeks. Strain out peels. Mix infused vinegar with an equal amount of water and place in a spray bottle to use.

Sink and Tub Scrub

1 cup baking soda

½ cup Castile soap

5 to 10 drops of antibacterial essential oil

(lavender, tea tree, rosemary)

Put baking soda in a bowl. Slowly add Castile soap, stirring continuously. Should be the consistency of frosting. Add essential oil and mix thoroughly. Store in airtight container.

To use: Scoop onto sponge and scrub surfaces, rinse. If more power is needed, add a little borax powder to surface before rinsing and wait 5 minutes. Should come sparkly clean.

Powder Cleanser

2 cups borax

1 cup baking soda

½ cup citric acid

½ cup kosher salt

20 drops lemon essential oil

Note: Although borax is natural, it can be toxic when ingested and should be kept away from children and pets. If you are concerned about using borax, you can omit it.

Combine all ingredients into a large bowl and stir until combined. Store in a large shaker bottle. To use, dampen surface and sprinkle powder over area you want to clean. Let sit for 15–30 minutes. For an extra cleansing boost, spray distilled vinegar on powder and wipe clean.

Tip: Use an old spice or Parmesan cheese container as your shaker bottle.

Tile Cleaner

1 cup white vinegar

Baking soda or salt

Heat vinegar and pour into spray bottle. Spray surface and wait 15 minutes. Dampen sponge or rag with vinegar and sprinkle with soda or salt. Rub down surface to remove film and scum. Rinse thoroughly.

Floor Cleaner For No-Wax Floors

1 cup white vinegar

¼ cup washing soda

2 gallons hot water

Combine ingredients, stirring until soda is dissolved. Mop as usual.

Laminate Floors

2 tablespoons white vinegar

1 quart warm water

Combine ingredients in a spray bottle. Spray floor in small sections and mop with a microfiber mop. Do not overspray as water may damage the floor. Or use in the canister of a spray mop.

Homemade Furniture Polish

You can use commercially prepared lemon oil. You can also make a simple polish by combining ¼ cup vinegar with ¾ cup olive oil and use a soft cloth to distribute the mixture over furniture. For wood furniture (or as an alternative to the first recipe), combine ¼ cup lemon juice with ½ cup olive oil, then follow the same procedure. Pour it on a soft cloth and work it into the wood, wiping with the grain. Buff till shiny.

Homemade Oxy-type Cleaner Recipe

2 tablespoons water

1 tablespoon hydrogen peroxide

1 tablespoon washing soda

Combine all ingredients and place in a sprayer to pre-treat stains or add to laundry and put on soak cycle for 30 minutes. Don't store this mixture as it loses effectiveness. Make only what you need at the time.

DIY Toilet Tablets

2 cups of baking soda

1-2 tablespoons of white distilled vinegar

1/2 cup of citric acid

35 drops of essential oils (example: 15 drops citrus and 20 drops of a "thieves"-type oil)

Mix baking soda and citric acid together into a large bowl. Add the vinegar into the baking soda mixture a couple of drops at a time, whisking between each addition. This is time consuming, but you really do need to go slowly. Add just enough vinegar to the mixture where you can form it into a clump with your hands. Add in the essential oils, mixing well to combine. Scoop the mixture into each section of a silicone ice cube tray and pack it firmly. Let the tablets set in the trays for at least an hour or longer. When they are completely hard, carefully pop each one out.

Notes:

Add in the Vinegar VERY Slowly - You want to add the vinegar 2 drops at a time. If you add it too quickly, your toilet tablets will not be as *fizzy*.

To Use - Drop one large tablet or two small tablets into the toilet bowl, let it dissolve completely. Then scrub it around with a toilet brush. At this point you can flush it away if you think it's done its work. Or if your toilet is needing it extra bad, let it sit for 30 minutes, then flush.

To Store - Store your toilet cleaner tablets in an airtight container so that they keep their strong scent.

Another DIY Toilet Tablet

1 cup baking soda

¼ cup cream of tartar

2 tablespoons hydrogen peroxide

20 drops essential oil of choice (lavender?)

To Make: Combine baking soda and cream of tartar in a large glass mixing bowl. Gradually add hydrogen peroxide, stirring in one tablespoon at a time. Add essential oil and stir to combine.

Spoon into silicone ice cube molds and press firmly to form to the molds. Place in a dry cool spot to set four to six hours. Gently pop tablets out of molds and store in a glass jar.

To Use: Place one tablet in the toilet and allow to completely dissolve for about 10 minutes before swishing with a brush and flushing. Use two to three times per week.

Goodbye to Dust Mites and Hello to a Cleaner Mattress

Most people spend around eight hours every night on their mattress and are completely unaware that they could be sharing their bed with millions of dust mites.

Dust mites are tiny bugs that are so small they can only be seen with a microscope. They stay alive by eating human skin flakes and thrive in a warm and humid environment. Ideal environments for dust mites usually include mattresses, pillows, carpets, upholstered furniture, and fabric-covered items. Dust mites can even cause an allergic reaction in some individuals that is similar to hay fever and asthma, making it difficult to breathe, or can even cause sneezing or a runny nose.

A simple way to rid dust mites is to clean your mattress, carpet, and upholstered furniture using just baking soda and essential oils.

Dust mites can be killed by using peppermint, eucalyptus or wintergreen essential oil. When combined with baking soda, which absorbs moisture, deodorizes and sanitizes, this powerhouse duo can be an extremely effective, natural, and non-toxic household cleaner.

What You Need:

1 cup baking soda (enough for a queen size mattress)

10 drops essential oil - *Lavender, Eucalyptus, Peppermint, Clove, or Rosemary*

Mason jar with lid

Sifter

Vacuum

How to:

1. Remove bed linens and wash them in hot water.

2. Add the baking soda and essential oils to a Mason jar. Shake to evenly distribute the oils.

3. Put the baking soda mixture into the sifter and sift across your mattress. *(You may need to double your baking soda mixture depending on the size of your mattress).*

4. Leave the mixture on your mattress for at least an hour. The longer you leave it, the better the results.

5. Once the mixture has been on the mattress for at least an hour, use your vacuum hose to remove the mixture from the mattress.

6. Make your bed with clean sheets and enjoy the fresh smell of your mattress. Repeat every 2-3 months, or as often as needed.

To deep clean your carpet or upholstered furniture, mix together the baking soda and essential oils and sift onto whatever area you are cleaning. Let it sit for at least one hour and then vacuum. It's easy—and effective!

Resources

Websites

https://www.motherearthliving.com/

https://www.nccih.nih.gov/health/herbsataglance

https://www.ewg.org/

https://womensvoices.org/

https://joybileefarm.com/

https://learningherbs.com/herbal-remedies/

https://thelostherbs.com/

https://www.anniesremedy.com/nccih.nih.gov/health/herbsa
taglance

https://blog.mountainroseherbs.com/

https://pubmed.ncbi.nlm.nih.gov/12730411/medlineplus.go
v/drugsinfo/herb

https://altnature.com/thelostherbs.com

https://pubmed.ncbi.nlm.nih.gov/anniesremedy.com

https://pubmed.ncbi.nlm.nih.gov/24354189/

https://www.ncbi.nlm.nih.gov/pmc/articles/PMC6271178/

https://www.tandfonline.com/doi/full/10.1080/19476337.20
17.1410499

https://simplelifemom.com/

https://www.ewg.org/news-insights/news-release/spring-
cleaning-ewgs-tips-what-use-and-what-avoid

https://www.ewg.org/ewgverified/cleaning-products.php

https://www.ewg.org/guides/cleaners/notices/20

https://www.epa.gov/greenerproducts/identifying-greener-
cleaning-products

https://brendid.com/natural-homemade-lemon-cleaning-products/

https://homeguides.sfgate.com/olive-oil-polish-hardwood-floors-105857.html

https://www.thespruce.com/uses-for-dish-soap-1900397

https://homeguides.sfgate.com/alcoholbased-recipe-hardwood-floor-cleaner-105487.html

https://www.bobvila.com/articles/ammonia-uses/

https://www.apartmenttherapy.com/borax-uses-cleaning-home-36659233

https://www.bhg.com/homekeeping/house-cleaning/cleaning-products-tools/homemade-cleaners/

https://www.apartmenttherapy.com/cleaning-floors-with-vinegar-265641

http://www2.epa.gov/saferchoice/safer-ingredients

https://greenseal.org/momremedy-on-changing-the-way-families-clean/

Publications

The Herbal Apothecary, 2015, JJ Pursell

Culinary Herbs for Short Season Gardeners, 2001,
    Ernest Small, Grace Deutsch

Herbs & Spices, 2002, Jill Norman

Herbs for Northern Gardens,1992, Dave Sands

Journal of Nutrition, May 2003;133(s):1286-90

Magazines

Herb Gardening, Meredith National Media Group

Better Homes & Gardens Herbs, 2021 Meredith
National Media Group

Herb Quarterly, 2020-2021, EGW Publishing

Made in the USA
Columbia, SC
12 May 2025

57601448R00093